# THE BODY AND BANK CONNECTION

## How to Exercise Your Way to Financial Fitness

# RITCHIE NKANA

10-10-10
Publishing

# DEDICATION

I dedicate this book to Janet and Henry. You both have had such a positive impact on my life. I share this dedication with Rico and Rochelle, for giving me clarity of reason.

# Table of Contents

# ACKNOWLEDGMENTS

Thank you to **Rico**, **Chel** and **Ruth**, for your patience and unfailing support.

To my family—**Zebina**, **Dafulin**, **Sabina**, **Nick**, **Judyn**, **Chuck**, **Maria**, and **Aries**—thank you for being incredible role models.

I am so thankful to you **Romnick**, for using your expert skills and creativity to breathe life into my ideas.

Thank you to my coaches and mentors, **Craig Ballantyne, Kerry Bartley, Carol McLachlan, Steve Foy, Vitor Fernandes, Ron Mourra**. You helped me see my potential and molded me into the leader I am today.

**Andreah**, you have been amazing, and this book would not have come to life without you.

Finally, I want to acknowledge my friends for all the support you have given me over the years, and for allowing me to bounce my many ideas off of you.

# FOREWORD

Are you living a life of physical health? Do you feel that you are financially free and on track to achieving your goals? Do you wish you could wake up every day feeling like your most productive self? Or, do you wake up every morning feeling exhausted and worried?

If you answered *yes* to that last question, you are not alone. Perhaps you are like so many other people, who spend every single day of their lives wishing that they were healthier, wealthier, and happier. The good news is you can be. You can have all of the abundance you desire; you simply have to commit. Commit to doing the work to change your daily habits, and you will see almost instant improvement.

You picked up this book because you are ready to do the work, and you are ready to see results. I am here to tell you that you are exactly where you need to be. Ritchie Nkana has developed a simple yet effective method that ties the work you do on your physical health with the work you do on your financial health. I know for a fact that you will be grateful that you have this book to guide you.

From his own experiences, Ritchie developed the *Body and Bank Connection* to help you achieve what he has achieved. His own personal transformation story is proof that his theories are correct, and that you can achieve your fitness and financial goals, at any stage in your life. When you realize that the work you are doing on your physical health can also be done with your financial health, you make the goal accessible. You give yourself the gift of efficiency. You take all of the complication out of it. You simplify what may at this moment feel like an unreachable goal, making everything possible.

Ritchie shares an easy to follow formula in a way that is fun to read. You'll get excited to wake up each day and work on your own personal development. His years of experience working with clients have allowed him to cultivate a greater understanding of your needs, and he is generous in sharing that knowledge with you.

Get ready to read this incredible journey and to embark on one of your own. You are here. It's time to free yourself from worry. It's time to feel energized. It's time to live a life of wealth and ultimate health!

Raymond Aaron
New York Times Bestselling Author

# Chapter 1

# WHAT IS THE BODY AND BANK CONNECTION?

**"It's not how much you earn
but what you do with what you earn."
—Jim Rohn**

This is so true! I was the victim of the never ending desire for a higher income for the longest time. Everything in my life depended on it.

*When I have a higher income I will be happy.*

*When I have a higher income I will focus on having meaningful relationships in my life.*

*When I have a higher income I will get in shape.*

*When I have a higher income I will go on adventures and truly experience the world.*

This is what I would tell myself. Does any of this sound familiar to you?

The result of this never ending desire to make more money was that everything else in my life took a back seat, including both my physical and mental health. I wasn't happy. I was constantly tired. I felt like I was running a race that didn't have an end in sight.

I began to question my daily choices. If I wasn't happy now, when would I be happy? Reflecting on my life, I knew I was doing well financially. I remembered back to when I first started out. I had far surpassed some of my earlier financial goals. And then the aha moment came: I realized I would never be happy with my income. There would always be a next level. There would always be more money to be made. It would never end, and that "one day" I was always working towards would never come.

I had to get off the hamster wheel and take a good look at my life. It began by taking a good, hard and honest look at my daily habits. Life didn't need to be about money for me to reach my financial goals. The truth of it is that making money isn't about money at all. Yes, you should educate yourself and take action based on that knowledge, but true financial freedom is achieved when you focus on your habits. Once I knew this and decided to take action on it, my life changed forever.

As I became more physically fit and healthy, I noticed a direct correlation to my financial fitness. The better I felt about myself, the more money I had in the bank. It was incredible. The shift within myself to change my habits, shifted every single aspect of my life. This is what I am here to share with you in this book. My practice is based on 5 simple pillars. Once you master these, you too will have the skills to transform your physical, emotional, and financial health.

Do I believe you can excel even if you aren't physically fit? Of course I do! There are many examples of people out in the world who are doing exactly that. But I believe they are not living at the most optimal level. When you achieve balance in your body and mind, you can achieve so much more!

## About Me

I've always set a high standard for myself. I believe that I am here for a purpose, and I know what that purpose is. I find it hard watching friends, family, colleagues, and clients struggle to gain control of their finances. We have created a culture of debt, which leaves most of us feeling stressed 99% of the time. But I believe it doesn't have to be this way. The more people who aren't living pay check to pay check and depending on credit cards or loans for larger purchases, the better off we will all be.

My love for numbers led me to becoming an accountant, for obvious reasons. I was ambitious and loved what I did, which is also why I hit that unhealthy point in my life when I knew I needed to change because I had become an overweight, burnt out accountant and entrepreneur who couldn't get out of bed in the morning.

I held onto some of the challenges I faced in life as excuses, in order to allow myself to continue with my unhealthy lifestyle. I had torn my achilles tendon while running, and my frustration over not being able to work out led me to being inactive and overweight. The other challenge I faced was time. I was young and a driven entrepreneur, who at the time was living pay check to pay check.

But one day I was done. I was done with all of the excuses I had been telling myself. If I wanted to get my health back on track and ultimately achieve the success I had been working towards, I had to make the time.

I've heard this from so many other busy parents, entrepreneurs and high-powered executives: "I just don't have the time to work out every day."

I know. I hear you. I was there. Like I said, I was too busy focused on achieving to take the time out of my day. It just wasn't important to me, until I realized it had to be. Does any of this sound familiar to you? What excuses are you telling yourself that are holding you back from achieving physical and financial success?

Take those excuses and allow them to tailor your approach to your health. For example, when you feel like you don't have time, combine one of your daily activities with exercise. If you have an injury, let it guide your approach to how you move your body. This is exactly what I did, and the journey it took me on led me to create Body & Bank Vitality.

I could feel my health holding me back. There are some pre-existing health conditions that run in my family, and they scared me. I realized I needed to take control, which meant making time and finding a way around my injury. I went on a mission to discover the best way to:

1.   Pull myself out of depression.

2.   Get back into healthier habits through moving.

3.   Find a workout that was both safe and efficient.

This journey led me to discovering metabolic training, and my life was forever changed. This type of training allowed me to train efficiently, and my sports therapist training ensured that the workouts were safe, efficient, and effective. I combined the principles of sports therapy with the efficiency principles of Metabolic Conditioning.

As I got healthier and fitter, my bank account grew. I realized that I could apply the same principles, that I had been using to get physically fit, to my finances. Ever since, I have been on a journey to help busy professionals and parents attain peak performance fitness without spending hours in the gym or on crash diets. And I combined financial transformation coaching based on the key idea that neglecting your health/fitness in order to chase financial freedom is counterintuitive. You can actually do both, and it will be even sweeter getting on the financial fitness journey when you fit in your body.

Body & Bank Vitality is a blueprint that brings together your physical and financial fitness. I combined my knowledge of finance with my knowledge of the body and coach my clients in both physical fitness and financial fitness, because I believe they are connected. In fact, I don't just believe it, I know it. I've lived the transformation.

- Physical energy is the foundation upon all energies, as espoused in the book *The Power of Full Engagement.* In this book, Jim Loehr and Tony Schwartz perfectly articulate how it's energy that drives performance, and is the foundation stone of the 4-tiered energy pyramid.

When I first decided to try to get healthier, I began by running. I soon realized that this wasn't right for my body. I began to feel the impact of it, and knew I needed to find another workout that was safe for my body. This is when I discovered metabolic conditioning, and my whole approach to fitness changed. It was as if something just clicked and I knew I had found the workout that was right for me. I am now a certified metabolic coach and certified sports therapist, helping others achieve what I have.

Everything changed, once I designed the program that was right for my life, and every single day I reap the rewards of being in the best physical and mental shape of my life. I help my clients to do the same. I've completely transformed my own life by changing my own daily habits, and I will never look back. This is living!

## The Mind/Body Connection

**"The mind is just like a muscle—the more you exercise it, the stronger it gets and the more it can expand."**
**—Idowu Koyenikan**

As an ambitious young accountant, I overlooked one very important aspect of the human body: everything is connected. Your body is so much more than simply a vehicle for your mind. All of it works together, and so when you are ignoring one, it will inevitably impact the other. This is the basic principle behind all that I do: your body and your brain are connected, and so are your physical fitness and your finances. When you work on both you give yourself the tools you need to reach even higher than you can imagine, in a shorter period of time.

So, how do you start? Sometimes making huge lifestyle changes can leave you feeling overwhelmed or even fearful of failure. Yes, it is easy to get home from work and unwind with a good show on Netflix and your junk food of choice, but over time this choice will make your life harder. The change from falling back into these comfortable daily habits is all about mindset.

*Mindset* is a word that is used so often in the self-development industry. The reason why every coach you will ever meet talks about it: mindset is everything. Shift your perspective and everything changes. Train your mind to believe you can achieve all you desire and you won't be able to ignore your needs any longer. When you have a mindset for growth, you will begin to develop healthier habits. I personally can't even imagine going back to my old way of being. Knowing what I do now, and having lived a more fulfilling life every single day, it would be impossible for me to go back to old limiting habits.

How then do you shift your mindset? This begins with understanding your big WHY. When you know and understand what your purpose is, it is difficult to stray off course. Your *why* is what guides each and every day. But the trick is, you have to be honest with yourself about your *why*. When you allow yourself to believe it is something it's not, before long you will begin to realize that something isn't right.

For example, in the beginning of my career I told myself again and again and again that my *why* was to achieve financial freedom. And yes, this is still a part of my *why*, but it only touches on a very small part. When I thought this was my whole *why*, I kept pushing, and nothing was ever good enough. So I worked harder and depended on my self-destructive habits for "self-care" when it was actually making me more tired. Following that *why* led me to burn out, which ultimately led me to discover my authentic, truthful *why*: to develop a program that will help myself as well as others achieve physical and financial health.

## Quick Exercise Break

Open up a new note on your phone or a new document on your computer, or turn the page in your journal and write out your *why*. Once you're done don't look at it again until you've finished reading this book. Reflect on the changes, if there are any. How did your *why* change? Why did your *why* change?

Back to my *why* . . . It wasn't until I understood the connection between my body and my mind that I was able to be honest with myself about my big *why*. I had originally thought that my path to achieving my financial goals was a straight one. Work hard and climb the corporate ladder and I would get there. I didn't waste time on anything else. But when I did start making my health a priority, it wasn't a waste of time and actually proved to keep me even more on track with my goal. A healthy body equals a healthy mind, and a healthy mind equals a healthy body. Taking it a step further: physical fitness equals financial fitness.

## The Body Vitality Solution

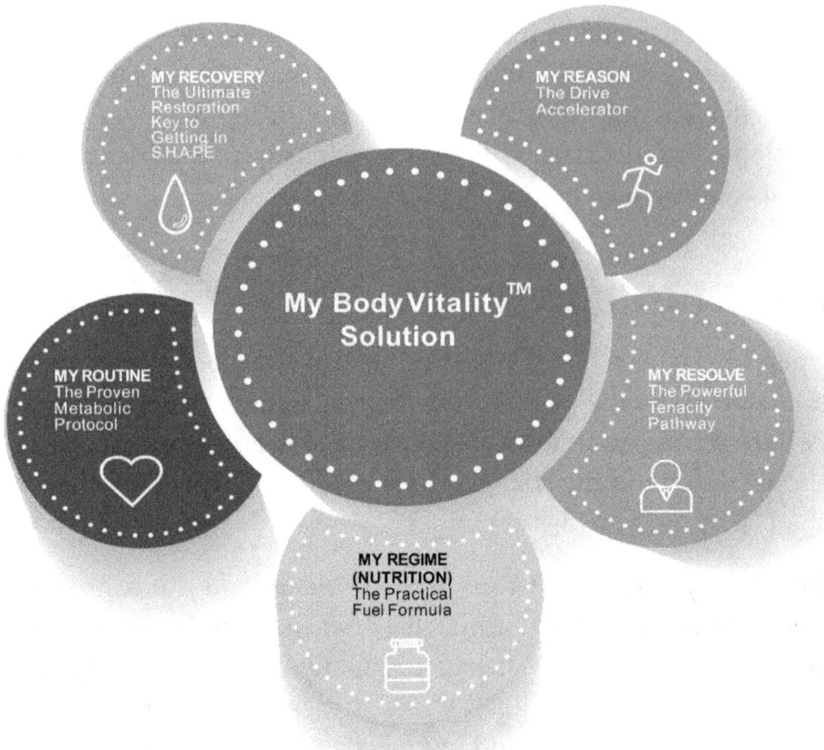


In the last section I shared with you one of the pillars of The Body Vitality Solution. I did so in order to give you context for the development of my roadmap, which involves five pillars in total.

Five pillars are:

1. Reason
2. Resolve
3. Regime
4. Routine
5. Recovery

I developed this program over the last decade of experience with my own training, as well as with my clients. I know this roadmap works because I've felt it and I've witnessed it. Each pillar is important to its efficacy, and so throughout this book I will dive more deeply into each; but for now, I'd like to give you a brief overview of the whole program.

## Your Reason

Your reason is what I refer to as the Dynamic Drive Accelerator. What is your big motivator? Getting to the root of why you are choosing to get involved in a fitness program will be the thing that will get you up and help you stick to the plan.

To determine why you are engaging into a fitness program, your bigger *why* has to be established. I know you already wrote out what you thought your *why* was. Ignore that. Right now, begin to get to the root of your bigger *why* by asking yourself the following questions:

1. **WHAT?**

   What are your goals?
   Do you want to lose weight?
   Do you want to gain muscle?
   Do you want to achieve better health?

2. **WHY?**

   Why do you want to achieve your goals?
   Is it so that you can achieve a more balanced lifestyle?
   Do you want to feel better about yourself so that you can be more confident in all areas of your life?

3. **WHERE?**

   Where are you at now?
   Where do you want to go?

4. **WHEN?**

   Set a date for achieving your goal.

Finally, how do all of these inform your big WHY? Could it be that you have an incredible story to share and you want to feel better about yourself so that you can gain the confidence to speak on large stages? Whatever your big WHY is, it needs to be important to you. Maybe your goal is to get healthy so that you can play more with your children, which informs your bigger WHY—to be a great mother or father figure, which again speaks to an even bigger WHY—to inspire others by leading them through the example you set with your actions.

Get in tune with your big WHYs and give yourself the Dynamic Drive Accelerator you need to keep you going on the tough days.

## Your Resolve

**"Resolve never to quit, never to give up, no matter what the situation."**

**—Jack Nicklaus**

I have developed something called The Powerful Tenacity Pathway. This is the support system that is going to give you everything you need to succeed.

Do you know why New Year's Eve resolutions usually don't work? Because people don't really mean it. The new year feels like a new start, and so it feels good to try to tackle some of the goals they want to achieve. It feels good to say you're going to make the changes you've always wanted to make in your life, but when it comes to actually making those changes, you haven't given yourself the tools you need to succeed.

I'm not saying you shouldn't make a New Year's resolution; all I'm saying is that if you do, resolve to see it through. Resolve to not give up, no matter how hard it is. Then give yourself the tools you need to succeed.

Use your strong *why* to help you to commit to a fitness program, backed up by social support and accountability. In my program I call these tools the 4 Cs. You might be starting to notice a pattern with the lettering of my lists. It's a tool I've given to my clients to help them easily remember what they need to succeed.

The 4 Cs of my coaching program are:

## 1. Commitment

Begin by committing to a 30 day challenge. There is much argument out there about the length of time it takes to make an action a habit. I don't worry much about the exact number, but I do think that committing to 30 days to start, rather than a shorter time, helps you get through some of the hurdles you'll encounter in your earlier days. It also gives you time to begin to really see how the changes begin to impact your life.

## 2. Challenges

At the beginning of your first month, write down at least three challenges you know you will face. For example, will you feel worried about the time commitment? Or, will your need for immediate success get in the way of your mindset? Whatever it is, accept, address it, and think about what will help you get through it. Do you need some positive affirmations for your mindset? Whatever it is, give yourself what you need!

## 3. Coaching

Congratulations! You've started with this book, which is the perfect place to get you excited about the changes you want to make and to give you some of the tools you need; but it is always good to get help. We are always better together. Join a coaching group or seek out 1-2-1 coaching.

### 4. Changes

You will feel the impact of the changes you are making right away. Some of them may feel negative at first. If you have looked forward to an alcoholic beverage every night after work, you may feel the social impact of not meeting up with your colleagues. If you use unhealthy food to calm your nerves, you may feel anxious when you can't have that food. But as time goes on, those feelings will ease and lead to even better feelings. Your mind will be clearer. Your body will feel better. You'll be excited to get up in the morning. You will be embracing the lifestyle changes.

This is the type of support system that is going to give you the accountability to commit to the program for your success.

## Your Routine

The Proven Metabolic Protocol is the routine you need to stay on track and motivated to keep on going! Combine your *why* with a nutritional plan and strategic exercises, and watch your body achieve its ultimate vitality. When this happens you will experience success in all areas of your life, including your finances. Your habits build your routine, and when you employ healthy habits in all areas of your life, you will succeed in all areas.

The workouts that you will do are different from others because they:

1.  are short and effective
2.  allow you to experience what is referred to as Afterburn or EPOC
3.  include time for recovery
4.  can be done anywhere

The Afterburn or EPOC refers to the elevation in metabolism (rate that calories are burned) after an exercise session ends. The increased metabolism is linked to increased consumption of oxygen, which is required to help the body restore and return to its pre-exercise state (Which means you could be burning calories 48 hours after your workout)

## Your Recovery

This is such an important step. It's the self-care you need to let your body rest before asking it to work hard for you again. Have you ever had a boss that asked so much of you, and never recognized your hard work with a bit of downtime at the end of a long, hard project? As soon as one project was complete, the next was right there waiting, with too much work to get done in too little time.

How good was that relationship? I would argue that over time you began feeling resentful, tired and unhappy with your daily life. I imagine you'd eventually quit and move on to a career that was more balanced.

If you treat your body in the same way as that boss who piled on the work, it's going to want to quit too. It'll start to break down, and refuse to do the things you need it to do. Keep your body working for you with this easy recovery method:

**The Ultimate Restoration Key to Getting in S.H.A.P.E:**

**S** LEEP

7 to 8 hours a sleep a night is optimal. Prioritize sleep. If you have to get up at 7am, start prepping for bed at 10pm. I know this sounds early if you're a night owl, but trust me, it is worth it and your body will thank you.

**H** YDRATE

Listen to your body and give it the water it needs. If you are thirsty, you've already deprived your body of hydration.

Generally I recommend 2-3 liters of water a day for women and 3-4 liters for men.

### **A** IR

Get outside! Seriously. Also, think about the air quality in your home. Is there anything that can be done to make it better? Open some windows? Buy an air purifier? Have more plants?

### **P** ERIOD

This is the rest period between workouts. It's an important aspect to the routine, as muscle growth and recovery happen when you rest.

### **E** NERGY

This is the end goal of implementing the 5 pillars to gain energy or vitality to enhance peak performance/productivity.

### What is Financial Fitness?

I define financial fitness as the progressive realization of your financial freedom by engaging in daily habits or disciplines that put you on the right trajectory to financial freedom.

To end this chapter, let's talk about financial freedom. It means something different to everyone. For some it means being able to afford life's necessities without worry. For others it means not living pay check to pay check. For some it means controlling your finances rather than having them control you, and for others it means owning a home and being able to travel.

For me, financial freedom meant being in control of my finances. In many ways, my finances controlled me when I was that ambitious accountant who could never have enough. The desire for more had me running the hamster wheel on full speed, with little time for self-reflection. I was so tired that my way of relaxing, in what little time I did have, was to zone out on the couch and feed my need for more with food. In every way, my desire for more "financial freedom" was controlling all of my actions.

It wasn't until I got off that hamster wheel and took control of my physical health that I was able to take control of my finances. When the realization hit me, it was like a lightbulb going off in my head. More like it exploded, actually. As I felt better, I did better at work, and there was more money in my bank account. It happened as I worked on myself.

Good physical fitness = financial fitness.

I am living proof that it is possible. As you move forward with this book, always keep in mind that in order to accelerate your goals you need to block out any bad energy, and anything that hinders you from reaching those goals. We are going to do that together.

Today is the day! Think about one thing that is stopping you. Whatever that thing is, recognize it and let it go. YOU CAN DO THIS! I am here to help every step of the way. This is my big WHY. Upgrading my health changed my life in such a big way. I am not only physically fit; I am also financially fit!

I've created a free clarity tool to help you keep track of your goals and your progress. You can download it on my website: www.bodyandbankconnection.com.

## What is Body Fitness/Vitality?

This is the vitality that enhances the physical, physiological and cognitive aspects of your being. This requires nurturing, and is not a destination but an ongoing process just like fueling your body with food. We just don't eat once and get filled up for good, but rather we have to continuously nourish our bodies. The same holds true when it comes to fitness.

# Chapter 2

# WHAT IS BODY FITNESS?

**"Nothing can stop the man with the right mental attitude from achieving his goal; nothing on earth can help the man with the wrong mental attitude."**
**—Thomas Jefferson**

At the end of the last chapter we looked at the definition of body fitness:

*This is the vitality that enhances the physical, physiological and cognitive aspects of your being. This requires nurturing, and is not a destination but an ongoing process just like fueling your body with food. w\We just don't eat once and get filled up for good, but rather we have to continuously nourish our bodies. The same holds true when it comes to fitness.*

As you might have noticed, there is so much more to body fitness than the physical aspect. In this chapter we are going to explore how your cognitive behaviors, your mood, your energy, your health, and your focus can all either help or hinder your overall body fitness. And not only that; we will also look at how these can be enhanced by better body fitness.

## Cognitive Behavior

**"People who exercise have better mental fitness, and a new imaging study from UC Davis Health System shows why. Intense exercise increases levels of two common neurotransmitters—glutamate and gamma-aminobutyric acid, or GABA—that are responsible for chemical messaging within the brain."[1]**

It has been proven time and time again that physical activity can improve cognitive functionality, especially in children and older adults. When you exercise you not only feel better physically, but also mentally. Think about how you feel in a day when you've been active. If you've gone on a long hike in the fresh fall air, or taken a yoga class for the first time in a long time. I imagine you'll say you feel better. I also imagine you might have slept better that night too.

It's easy to see how exercise helps you feel better mentally. You might also feel a sense of accomplishment for having taken the time to do something you've wanted to do for so long. You might feel a diminished sense of guilt for having neglected your own health. You might feel better about yourself, and have a heightened sense of confidence, knowing that you are taking control of your health. All of these things are normal, and I'll talk more about how they have a positive effect on your mood a little later in the chapter.

For now, however, I want to address how exercise is being using to battle depression and other neuropsychiatric disorders. These disorders are linked with deficiencies in neurotransmitters, which help our brain communicate to our body when we are feeling both emotionally and physically healthy.

"Major depressive disorder is often characterized by depleted glutamate and GABA, which return to normal when mental health is restored," said study lead author Richard Maddock, professor in

---

[1]  https://www.sciencedaily.com/releases/2016/02/160225101241.htm

the Department of Psychiatry and Behavioral Sciences. "Our study shows that exercise activates the metabolic pathway that replenishes these neurotransmitters."[2]

I don't want us to get too bogged down in the science here, so basically what I'm trying to say is that moving your body does so much more than simply lift your mood; it is integral to how you live your life, every moment of every day. Yes, you might be thinking you are doing great right now. You make good money, you have a nice home, and you have the ability to afford luxuries others don't. But imagine what you could do if your body wasn't running on empty. Imagine what you could do if your body was in its best shape. Imagine just how much more money you could make, or how much more impact you could have on the world around you if you were functioning at your most optimal.

When you think about it that way, it's hard to ignore the facts: your physical fitness is directly linked to your ability to perform at your highest level in all areas of your life. If you still don't believe me, let's look at a few more facts:

1. According to Richard Maddock, vigorous exercise is the most demanding activity the brain encounters, even more so than calculus or chess.

2. Regular exercise improves heart health and blood flow to the brain, making your cognitive functioning more focused, sharp, and clear.[3]

3. Exercise has the ability to lift your mood, which will inevitably improve workplace performance.[4]

---

[2] https://www.sciencedaily.com/releases/2016/02/160225101241.htm

[3] https://www.sciencedirect.com/science/article/pii/S105381192030985X

[4] https://hbr.org/2014/10/regular-exercise-is-part-of-your-job

In a study done by Leeds Metropolitan University with over 200 employees, they found that that their work experience changed on the days when they were able to visit the gym. They reported having more patience when challenges arose amongst team members, being able to manage their time better, and having clearer focus on the task at hand.

Two simple takeaways:

1.  Regular, vigorous exercise can help fight depression.
2.  Daily exercise can improve your overall performance not only at work but in all areas of your life.

I pulled this information from three articles which I've cited in the footnotes, in case you'd like to read more. But in all honesty you can find hundreds of thousands of articles on the subject that prove exactly these points. It is no secret that exercise improves our productivity. So why, then, is it so hard to prioritize regular physical activity into our lives? We know it because we feel it when we exercise. We know it because we feel it when we don't exercise. And yet, for many of us it can be the first thing to slip when we get "too busy."

Throughout this chapter, I am going to provide you with some mindset hacks to help you stay on your game and put your physical fitness at the top of your priority list. These are just some starter hacks to get you thinking about it. In chapter 4 we will dive deeper into mindset and how to set yourself up for success. For now, give these a try!

**Mindset Hack #1**

For this first mindset hack all you need to do is remind yourself that you are worth it. You are bigger than your goals. You are stronger than you think. And you can do anything you set your mind to.

Sometimes when we have let ourselves spiral down, it can be hard to change our habits. It's comfortable to do what we know.

It's easy to not try. This mindset hack is simple, easy and maybe just a little cliché. But it's okay to be cliché, and it's okay to feel a bit silly.

When you look in the mirror in the morning, say these three things:

I am awesome.
I am strong.
I can do this.

Feel free to modify these affirmations in any way. Make them sound like you. You can also write them out over and over again in a journal if that works for you. You can write them out and stick them on your mirror so you can read them whenever you need to.

If you'd like to dive deeper in this exercise, listen to your thoughts as you say, read, or write out these affirmations. Are they trying to prove you wrong? Our subconscious or even conscious thoughts can be tricksters. They want you to stay the same. Change is hard! Take control of these negative thoughts, that are doing their very best to reinforce limiting self-beliefs, by recognizing them and letting them go.

Not sure what I mean? Let me help. Sometimes as you think something like "I am strong," your mind will pull up memories to prove you wrong. As you speak the affirmation, you may experience a flash of a time when you failed at something and it made you feel weak. Recognize the memory and counter it with one where you showed your strength.

Taking control of your thoughts and moving beyond those beliefs that are stopping you from achieving optimal health is an incredibly powerful tool.

## Productivity

**"It's not always that we need to do more but rather that we need to focus on less."**

**—Nathan W. Morris**

When people say they don't have time, what they mean to say is that they don't have time to self-actualize. It's all about priorities! What do I mean by self-actualize? It's simple really: when you self-actualize, you accept yourself for who you are. When you do that, you do all that you can to be the very best version of yourself.

So, when someone says that they don't have time to take care of their physical fitness, what they are saying is that they don't have time to accept themselves and to prioritize their lives as a whole. When you ignore a portion of your own needs, you're prohibiting yourself from becoming your true self, and in doing so I feel that you are not accepting your best self. You are willing to settle for the lesser version of you, the version that might still be succeeding in life, but not in the way that you know you could be.

When you say you don't have time it means you're not willing to make time. But the key here is to understand that when you make the time to become physically fit, it impacts your productivity across the board.

What is the simple definition of productivity?

**pro·duc·tiv·i·ty**

**the effectiveness of productive effort, especially in industry, as measured in terms of the rate of output per unit of input.**

Yes, you might be productive, but could you be even more productive? Could one unit of your input equal a greater output rate? When you achieve full body fitness, the answer is always yes. You'll be able to put in less effort and achieve more success. Put in the effort for 20 minutes a day and watch how much more you achieve in all areas of your life while feeling more energized and fulfilled.

Less input = greater output! There is a direct correlation between how much you can achieve when you have clear, direct, and focused energy. Achieving full body fitness allows you to have that. But first things first, you have to get your priorities straight!

**Mindset Hack #2**

This hack is all about getting your priorities straight! Or more to the point, setting your priorities to be in alignment with your goals, no matter what they are. So, I've established that when you exercise you are more productive throughout the day. That said, if exercising for 20 minutes a day will increase your productivity throughout the day, doesn't it stand to reason that you will get more done in the 8-hour work day if you take 20 minutes to work out? You'll most likely get more done throughout the day than you would in the 20 minutes you would have if you choose to skip the workout.

Try this hack:

When you first wake up in the morning, before you get out of bed, imagine yourself having a great workout, and transition from that in your visualization to imagine yourself returning home from your work day having accomplished everything. Imagine the feeling of accomplishment. See yourself walking taller and with even more confidence.

If that nagging voice in the back of your mind is saying: "Just go straight to work. That extra half an hour will give you a leg up on the day," stop and remind yourself that it may allow you to get a few extra things done in the morning, but you will slow down throughout the day, ultimately being less productive overall. Come back to that visualization of yourself working out, and how good it is going to feel in the moment and at the end of the day when you've accomplished all that you set out to accomplish.

If you find the voice winning, pulling you back to old habits, simply say this:

**When my body is strong, I am strong.**
**When my body is strong, I am productive.**
**When my body is strong, my life is more fulfilling.**

## Energy

Energy feels like a simple concept to grasp, right? Some days you feel like you have more energy and some days you feel like you have less. Some people feel like, if they nourish their bodies with healthy foods and get enough sleep, they should have a good amount of energy. Of course, both of these things will help you have the energy you need to get through your day, but they are only addressing your physical body.

Your body is made up of four connected parts that all have their own energy, and needs. Those parts are: mental, spiritual, emotional, and physical. If you were to take a moment and look at your life now, how are you feeding all four of these areas of yourself? Are there some areas that could use a little more fuel?

As humans, we are all unique. Your needs are different from the person sitting beside you at the coffee shop. They are different from your life partner's. They are different from the stranger who has joined you for a zoom conference. How you fuel up yourself in these areas might be very different from anyone else, but the simple fact is that we all need fuel in all of them.

In this book, *The Power of Full Engagement*, Jim Loehr and Tony Schwartz famously proclaim that most of us are chasing the wrong resource: hours in the day. Instead, we should focus on something entirely different: our energy.

Our energy can be broken down into 4 different elements:

Your physical energy – how healthy are you?

Your emotional energy – how happy are you?

Your mental energy – how well can you focus on something?

Your spiritual energy – why are you doing all of this? What is your purpose?"[5]

When I think back to how I used to live before I had a radical shift in life to live as the best version of me, I know that I wasn't providing any of my four energy elements with the fuel they needed. At the time I might have argued that I was focused solely on feeding my spiritual energy—my purpose—because I was chasing my dream of having more and more money. But I wasn't even doing that, because ultimately money and financial freedom are not my actual *why*. Those goals may be a positive outcome from achieving my purpose, but they are not my purpose.

Now I look at the different ways I can help fuel all areas of myself.

To keep my physical energy up I do the following:

1.  I take care of my body by achieving a full body fitness.

2.  I make sure I get enough sleep.

3.  I am conscious of the food I eat and do my best to give my body the nutrients it needs.

4.  I take time to rest and renew my energy.

When I fuel my physical energy it is easier for me to fuel my mental, emotional, and spiritual energy. I have a base to pull from if the others are depleted. Having a strong physical energy can help

---

[5]  https://buffer.com/resources/the-4-elements-of-physical-energy-on-how-to-master-them/

me focus mentally, address my emotional needs in the moment, and understand when I have stepped out of integrity with my purpose. There are also ways I can build more energy spiritually, emotionally and mentally, but without that physical energy base I won't have what I need to push forward.

Some of the things I do now to achieve that base are:

1. **For my emotional energy**, I get quiet and check in with myself. What am I feeling? Why am I feeling these things? Is there a need for a perspective shift in my thought patterns?

2. **For my mental energy**, I keep on learning. The constant pursuit of new knowledge is one of the most effective ways to build our mental energy and keep it strong as we age.

3. **For my spiritual energy**, I continue to do the work to live in integrity with my purpose, my big WHY!

Where are you at now with your energy levels? Have you built a strong physical base from which to grow, or are you where I was years ago: chasing more time in the day to achieve a purpose that wasn't in alignment with my *why*?

Energy starts with motion; if we go back to Newton's first law of motion—an object at rest remains at rest and an object in motion remains in motion unless an outside force acts against it. This also applies to our body energy. You should not wait until you have a ton of energy before you can get started on a task, but rather you will find that when you get started that then builds up the energy required, and the motivation to push through and complete the task. As Earl Nightingale would say, you should not ask for heat then put the wood in the fire, but rather you should first put the wood in the fire, then you can get the heat.

## Your Health

Assessing your energy levels is a great place to start when it comes to understanding your deficiencies in all four areas. I believe we can view our health in the same way we view energy. When you have a healthy physical base you can easily achieve greater emotional, mental, and spiritual health. And this begins with getting fit!

When you are active, your body is healthier than it ever will be when you're not. That is a fact. YOU ARE HEALTHIER WHEN YOU ARE ACTIVE! The only way to build a strong base is to work on your physical being as a whole. This means, of course, being active, eating well, and listening to your body.

The definition of health is: the state of being free from illness or injury. The minute I read that, I thought, "Is that really right?" Health is simply the absence of something negative. I feel like the definition of health should be all about the positive. So I searched further, and found a definition from the WHO that felt better:

**Health** is a state of complete physical, mental and social well-being and not merely the absence of disease or infirmity.[6]

Even though this definition feels better to me, it still doesn't hit the mark. This is my definition of health: Being healthy means feeling good.

I wake up with energy. I'm ready to take on the day. My body feels alive with excitement. I live in the moment of my life and listen to my physical, mental, emotional, and spiritual needs. I am constantly growing and changing to meet those needs.

What is your definition of health? Take a moment now and write it down. As you write, think about where you are at now in terms of

---

[6]  https://www.who.int/about/who-we-are/frequently-asked-questions

achieving your optimal health. Give yourself a rating from 1 to 10; 10 being your best possible health and 1 being unhealthy.

Physical   – ① ② ③ ④ ⑤ ⑥ ⑦ ⑧ ⑨ ⑩
Mental   – ① ② ③ ④ ⑤ ⑥ ⑦ ⑧ ⑨ ⑩
Emotional – ① ② ③ ④ ⑤ ⑥ ⑦ ⑧ ⑨ ⑩
Spiritual   – ① ② ③ ④ ⑤ ⑥ ⑦ ⑧ ⑨ ⑩
Overall   – ① ② ③ ④ ⑤ ⑥ ⑦ ⑧ ⑨ ⑩

Here is a bit more information to help you:

**Physical** – You actively work on your physical fitness every day. This energizes you and lifts your energy.

**Mental** – You feel focused and are able to easily grasp new concepts.

**Emotional** – You are able to recognize, work through, and release the emotions that aren't serving you.

**Spiritual** – You know what your purpose is in life. You make decisions based on your WHY.

Throughout this book you will continue to work on all areas of your own personal health and wellness. Mark this page when you are done reading and come back to it. My hope for you is that your ratings will be higher, and maybe even your overall definition of what health means to you will have grown.

## Your Ability to Focus

**"The successful warrior is the average man, with laser-like focus."**

**—Bruce Lee**

I love those moments when my mind is clear and I can easily focus on the task at hand. I thrive in those moments, and they give me even more energy to achieve all that I want to in a day.

I experience more of those moments when I have achieved an overall body fitness. My mind is clear and I am at my best.

Think about the days when your body feels heavy and your thoughts are jumbled and cloudy. It takes longer to get anything done because your mind easily wanders off. Many of my clients have reported to me that on the days they take the time to work out before they head into the office, it is easier to focus. They get things done quicker and feel more productive throughout the day. Let this be your reminder: You will achieve more in the day if you take that 20 minutes for yourself and your body than you would if you skip it to head into the office early.

I know that it's easy to get distracted by shiny objects, like money. I've been there, and it led me down a very unhealthy path. I am back on track and here to tell you that you will have a healthier bank account when you have a healthier body.

As I was writing this chapter I did a quick search for tips on achieving a higher level of focus. The most common topics people address are removing distractions, and mindfulness. While I agree that being more mindful and setting up a distraction-free work zone are great tools, I believe the most important aspect of achieving great mental clarity is a healthy, active body. Your body is connected. It's not simply a vehicle for the brain. Your body informs your brain. Your body supplies your brain. Your body is your brain. Work on your body and you'll see a huge shift in how much you are able to focus.

## Your Mood

Your mood is connected to your ability to focus. When you exercise, your body releases chemicals called serotonin and dopamine. "Dopamine and serotonin are chemical messengers, or neurotransmitters, that help regulate many bodily functions. They have roles in sleep and memory, as well as metabolism and emotional well-being. People sometimes refer to dopamine and serotonin as the "happy hormones" due to the roles they play in regulating mood and emotion."[7]

A deficiency of either of these chemicals can lead to low mood or even depression. I know that it can be hard to pull yourself up and out of bed early to work out when you are feeling low. I also know that it can be hard to push yourself to work out if you've already put in a long day at work. We've all been there. We've all talked ourselves out of going to the gym because of our low mood.

The one thing I know for sure is that every single time I pushed past my desire to pull the blankets back over my head, and made it to the gym, I felt better. I felt better not only because of the dopamine and serotonin; I felt better because I made the tough choice and I succeeded. Before even going to the office, I had accomplished something for me, which made the rest of the day even easier, no matter what challenges I faced. Your mood will always be lifted by physical activity.

## Your Body Fitness

What is it that drives the conversation?

Let that question sit with you for a moment.

Not sure what I mean by conversation? That's okay. I am here to explain! The conversation is everything. The conversation with yourself. The conversation with your friends. The conversation with your colleagues. The conversation with your clients. The conversation with your children. The conversation with your boss.

---

[7]  https://www.medicalnewstoday.com/articles/326090

## WHAT IS IT THAT DRIVES THE CONVERSATION?

The answer is simple: Value.

I know this can be an odd way to think about simple conversations you have in life, but once you think about it a little more, you'll realize how true it is. Do you want to stick around for a conversation that isn't providing you value in the moment in some way? I would argue that you don't. Even if you are stuck, say at a dinner party with friends or at a presentation at work, if the conversation isn't holding your attention by providing some sort of value to your life, you'll let your thoughts wander.

The conversation we are having right now about your body fitness is providing immense value. Keep it going with yourself. Don't drop it. From chasing a never-reachable goal while feeling miserable and exhausted, to achieving greater success, financial freedom, and overall health, I am a living example of how this conversation changed my life completely. I keep the conversation about my body fitness going, every single day. Because it will always have value. My ability to stay active and healthy has an ongoing impact on my success in all areas of my life. This is why the system that I use works. 20 minutes of high impact exercise every single day doesn't take up too much time, and establishes a strong habit. If you are busy, that's okay . . . you have time for this!

# Chapter 3

# YOUR REASON

**"The goal is not simply for you to cross
the finish line, but to see how many people
you can inspire to run with you."
—Simon Sinek**

If you don't have a reason, you will never make it to the finish line. And that is not what I want for you. You have to know why you are doing something, or when the going gets tough it'll be super easy to quit.

When you have a reason and it is one you will fight for no matter what, you won't let yourself quit. You won't be able to let yourself because your reason is so important to you. If you were to let go of that reason you'd be devastated; it would be as if you removed an arm. This is why I call your reason the dynamic drive accelerator.

It is DYNAMIC because it is ever-evolving. It shifts and changes as you grow.

It DRIVES you because it makes you hungry. Your reason is the one thing that has your back no matter what. It's the biggest fan you've got in your cheering section. It wants you to succeed because when you succeed it continues to exist. Your reason both depends on you for life, and gives you life.

It ACCELERATES your growth because it asks you to push yourself to succeed. Your reason gives you momentum.

Begin your work in this chapter by answering this question: Is your reason strong to be your dynamic drive accelerator? It should be so important, so big, so impactful, that you can't deny it. You can't possibly fail because your reason won't let you.

If your answer is YES without a shadow of a doubt, that is amazing. This chapter will ask you to understand that reason completely. If your answer is NO, that is 100% okay too. This chapter will ask you to keep working to uncover your reason and help you use it to push you forward towards your goals.

## Where Are You Now?

The best place to start is with acceptance. Accept yourself for where you are in this very moment. Stop blaming yourself for how you let yourself get here. It's a waste of time. How you got here doesn't matter anymore. It's how you move forward from here that is important. But first you must truly accept where you are.

Easier said than done. It can be hard to see what you don't really want to see, because when you see it, you can't un-see it. Ultimately at this point you then need to accept it. With acceptance comes a choice; you can either choose to ignore it or take on the responsibility to change it. I hope you have picked up this book because you either know you need to accept a truth about your current reality or you have already accepted that truth, and you are ready to take responsibility and change it. You are ready to jump in.

I remember the morning I woke up and knew I needed to accept that I was overweight, unhealthy, and unhappy. I woke up to the reality of what it felt like to live in my body every single day. I let the worry of what this was doing to my life expectancy and ability to truly achieve my goals wash over me. Rather than pushing them aside for another day, I let what I was doing to my body sink in.

I was slowly killing myself, and I had no one to blame but me. It wasn't the universe. It wasn't the history of heart issues that runs in my family. It wasn't the boss who pushed me too hard. It was me. I was making the choice to live each day in my obese body, and drown my worries over what I was doing to myself in work and unhealthy behaviors.

I woke up that morning and realized that I couldn't live that way anymore. I was done. Things needed to change. I didn't want to just get by anymore. I was more worried about my overall health. I was miserable. This was the day I accepted that I was obese, and took responsibility for my situation.

## Your Pain

Accepting where you are at means recognizing your pain. It means addressing it. It means feeling it. Now is the time to rip the bandaid off. You feel this pain every single day. Yet, you do your best to pretend that it's not hurting. You shove it down. You try not to think about it. You tell yourself that that is how the world is and there's nothing you can do about it.

GET REAL WITH YOURSELF! Yes, ripping the bandaid off and exposing your pain is going to hurt, but in the long run it is going to hurt a whole lot less than it will if you continue to live the way you are. So get real with yourself. Are you broke? Are you drowning in an ever-increasing sea of debt? Are you overweight? Are you so out of shape you can't make it up more than one flight of stairs without feeling it?

Be honest! Accepting your pain and taking ownership of your current reality provides you with a starting point on your GPS. This is where you are now, and that is 100% okay. What is not okay is allowing yourself to live in this pain. Living in this pain is not what the universe wants for you.

Peel the layers back on your pain. What is it doing to your life now? Many of my clients feel that their obesity is hurting their quality of life because they can't play with their children or grandchildren in the way they would like to. Or it is causing a feeling of exhaustion that makes everything a struggle. Sometimes these same clients also feel it has impacted their ability to achieve their career and financial goals as well. Their poor health is impacting their productivity in ways they never realized it would.

**The Look Back Exercise**

One of the things I love to do to help keep me on track with both my fitness and financial goals is to imagine myself a year from now if I don't take control of my pain. For example, if I were still overweight today and I didn't do anything at all about it, what would that look like in my life, and how would I feel looking back on myself today?

I know, I know . . . it's a bit confusing. Basically you are looking forward at yourself in 12 months to how that version of yourself would feel looking back on you today knowing that you made the choice to not do anything.

This exercise works best if you write it down. So sit down and open a new document on your phone or computer, or grab your journal and a pen. Ask yourself this:

1.  What is my current pain?

2.  If I don't do anything about my current pain what will my life be like in 12 months?

3.  As the version of myself who chose to do nothing, how
    will I feel about myself looking back on this moment?

Let me share a hypothetical example with you to get you started:

## 1. What is my current pain?

I am overweight now. It makes me feel so tired. I constantly
worry about having a heart attack at a young age like my
mother did. My knees ache when I walk up the stairs and
I can feel my mobility declining. I know that I need to take
the time to exercise and make healthier food, but I am just
so busy with work, I just don't feel like I can take the time.

## 2. If I don't do anything about my current pain what will my life be like in 12 months?

I am even heavier and having to take medication for my
high blood pressure. I am making the choice more and more
often to take the elevator or escalator. It feels difficult to
move my body and getting up in the morning takes so much
more energy. I know I want to change but it is even more
overwhelming. Although I have progressed in my career
(because it is one of the only aspects of my life I have given
priority to), it's not nearly as much as I had thought I would
be at this time. I am depressed. Even when I do achieve a goal
or do something I would normally love to do, I feel little joy.

## 3. As the version of myself who chose to do nothing, how will I feel about myself looking back on this moment?

Looking back on myself 12 months ago as the person who
knew there was a problem and did nothing about it, I feel
angry and ashamed. I am so mad at my past self for not
taking control because a year later I see not only how much
worse things have gotten, but how much I could've achieved
in that time, had I just started.

Take this exercise even further by looking ahead and back to five years from now and even ten years from now. How much harder? How much more overwhelming will it be to take control of your pain? Think about it like a house that has been filled with clutter over the years. When it first starts happening, there are some warning bells.

"Maybe I should organize and get rid of the clothes I don't need any more," you think to yourself. You've added the ones you think you don't want into garbage bags to make room in your closet, but you know you want to go through them again before donating them. But then you have something else more important to get done and so you add those bags to the storage room. You'll get to them soon. It won't take long. Or at least that's what you think as you shut the door and completely forget about those bags.

The next year, you decide to buy yourself new dishes for the kitchen, but you're not sure you want to just get rid of your old ones so you put them in a box and hide them away in your storage room. This pattern continues for another 5 years until that storage room that was once empty is now filled with stuff you haven't even looked at, from floor to ceiling. Now the task is big and will take days. You know you have to do it.

The weight of the stuff you don't need any more has been weighing on you. It's time to make it a priority, but when you look back on the version of yourself that simply added a few bags of clothing to a room and thought you'd get back to it, you with you hadn't ever established that pattern. You wish you would've taken the extra hour to try on all of the clothes, make your final decision and drive the unwanted items to the donation center.

The little task has now become one that will take days of your time. You regret your past decisions, but you don't let that bring you down. In five years, you know you want to look back on the person who today took control of the situation and eliminated the pain going forward.

## Discover Your Big Why

**"Do not wait; the time will never be just right. Start where you stand, and work with whatever tools you may have at your command, and better tools will be found as you go along."**

**—George Herbert**

Here you are: You've recognized the pain you are in, and you've accepted it. You've ripped the bandaid off. You've gotten real with yourself. It hurts. I know it does. And I am sorry to tell you there is no quick or easy fix. Don't let that get you down. Let it fuel you. Once you gain momentum on your goals you will feel so good. I've lived it and I've witnessed it again and again and again. Do the work. Put in the effort. You will never, ever regret it.

It's time to dive deeper into your big *why* to discover the reason you will stick to the changes you need to make in your life. Right now you might be thinking you know exactly what your *why* is. Maybe it feels simple: You want to be able to play with your children without getting tired.

YES! Of course that is a great *why*. But is this the BIG why? Is this your dynamic drive accelerator? It might be. Playing with your children just might be the thing to keep you going on those mornings when you'd rather get a jump start on your day at work, or you don't think you can pull yourself out of bed twenty minutes earlier. You are the only one who knows exactly what drives you, and we are all unique.

Even if you think you know without a doubt what your big *why* is, I am still going to ask you to complete this exercise with me. When I first embarked on my own fitness journey I believed my *why* was that I wanted to feel better. And I wasn't wrong. I did and I still do want to feel better, but that isn't my ultimate reason for embarking on the journey that I did. Wanting to feel better was a surface level *why*, but it was a great place to start.

To truly connect to my dynamic drive accelerator I needed to go levels deeper . . .

I use a very simple concept that many others have used before me. I simply continue to ask myself "why?" Just like that curious child who wants to know more, I keep pushing myself to get to the root of the truth—to get to the real reason I push myself to be the healthiest, happiest, and most successful version of myself.

You can do this too. I'll share with you an example of the **Layers Deep *Why*** exercise:

**What is your pain?**

My pain point is that I am overweight, out of shape, and worried about my health.

**Why do you want to heal this pain?**

I want to heal this pain so that I can feel better.

**Why do you want to feel better?**

I want to feel better for so many reasons, but I think the main reason is that I'd like to feel better about myself.

**Why do you want to feel better about yourself?**

I'd like to feel better about myself because it's terrible not liking how I look in the mirror. It's terrible loathing myself for not taking care of me.

**Why do you want to not loathe yourself?**

This seems like a no-brainer really. Who wouldn't want to like themselves?

**Okay . . . why do you want to like yourself?**

Because when I like myself I make healthier choices.

**Why do you want to make healthier choices?**

I want to make healthier choices because when I am healthy I am more productive.

**Why do you want to be more productive?**

When I am more productive I have a positive impact on the world around me.

**Why do you want to have an impact on the world around you?**

It is important for me to have a positive impact on the world around me because I believe I can use my knowledge to help others live more fulfilling lives.

**Why do you want to help others live more fulfilling lives?**

I want to help others live more fulfilling lives because when people are fulfilled they feel at peace, and when people are at peace they are kinder to those around them. I want to help make the world a kinder place.

I think you get the idea. Try this for yourself. Here is a little bit of advice if you get stuck:

1. Even if the answer feels basic, write it out.

2. There is no right or wrong.

3. Remember, you are not trying to be unique or smart or anything other than what you need to be.

4. If you think you're done after three questions, you're not . . . keep pushing.

5. As you keep peeling those layers you will feel it and it will become apparent when you hit your real underlying *why* . . .

6. Hold onto that why; it should be your anchor on days when you do not feel like getting out of bed to put in that workout, the driver to get you to put in that extra push-up when you thought you were done, or indeed even the catalyst to making that very first step to schedule half an hour a week to look at your finances.

Your *why* is huge! Take the time to really explore it. Understand it, and what it truly means to you. When you think you've gotten to the bottom layer, or at least the bottom layer for now, take a moment and reflect on what a day in the life of the version of you who is living in their *why* looks like.

Here's a quick example based on the answers from above:

*As the man who lives in my why each and every day, I open my eyes and before getting out of bed I set my intention for the day. I speak to myself: "I feel energetic today. I feel energetic today. I feel energetic today!"*

*I head to the gym for a short workout at 7:30. Once my workout is complete I meet with my first client of the day. The maximum amount of clients I serve in a day is 4. In each meeting I actively listen to their needs. I give them my full attention. My goal is that they leave feeling better for having worked with me that day.*

*I leave time every day for business growth and my own personal development. This could be either reading a book, having a call with my own coach, or taking a course. In the evening I spend time making a healthy meal to enjoy with family.*

What does a day in the life of the version of you who lives in their *why* look like? Are you excited when you think about it? If not, you may want to revisit your *why*. Is it possible that you've haven't gotten to the bottom layer? Is it possible that your reason for making the changes you crave isn't strong enough to hold you to your goals yet? Keep going! I know that reason is within you. If you still need help, I coach my clients through this exercise all the time. Check out my website for more information on what I do: www.bodyandbankconnection.com.

## The Fork in the Road

**"One of the most important things that I have learned in my 57 years is that life is all about choices. On every journey you take, you face choices. At every fork in the road, you make a choice. And it is those decisions that shape our lives."**

**—Mike DeWine**

Each and every single day you will be faced with a choice:

*Do you stay on your path, or do you veer off of it?*

Sometimes you have to veer off your path. Sometimes you need to revisit your reasons. But when your reasons are strong, and you truly know what is driving you, you'll never choose to turn down the road where there is never enough time for you to achieve your *why*-driven goals.

Have you ever heard of Parkinson's Law? Not to be confused with the neurodegenerative disorder, Parkinson's Law has to do with time and how you use it. According to wikipedia.org, Parkinson's Law is the adage that work expands so as to fill the time available for its completion.

So, you see, you always have enough time to do the things you make priority for. ALWAYS! When I incorporated working out into my everyday routine, everything got better. I was more efficient. I was more driven to succeed than I ever have been before. And I was driven to learn and grow in more ways than I thought possible for me.

## Your Drive to Learn

When connecting with your *why* you will ultimately be inspired to not only heal the pain you originally intended to heal, but to learn more about how you can be the best version of yourself in all areas of your life. This is inevitable.

Why? Have you ever noticed that when you have been working on being a better version of yourself, there are some people who just don't fit in your life anymore? It's not that they aren't worthy of you, or you feel like you're better than they are. They just don't fit. It could be the friend who is constantly trying to bring you back down to you your own unhealthy ways, or the family member who asks you, "Who do you think you are?!" You find yourself not wanting to be around them as much as you used to. You might choose a nice dinner out rather than an all-night binger with the boys.

It's kinda like that, but within the different aspects of yourself. When there is a part of you that isn't keeping up with the rest, you ultimately will crave to help it grow. You'll want to leave the old version of that aspect of you behind.

This is what I found with my own journey to better health, which ultimately led me to connecting my physical fitness shaping my money mindset. A few things happened here:

1.  The better I felt physically, the more energy I had. The more energy I had, the more efficient I was at work. The more efficient I was at work, the more money I made.

2.  I realized that my mindset around money was all wrong.

Although the first point is very important, if your goal is to gain greater health both physically and financially, beginning your workout routine will help you begin that part of your journey. But the second point is the one I want to finish up this chapter focusing on; in particular, how these same fitness principles can be applied as a starting point to your financial transformation journey. What are the reasons why you want to improve your finances? It all starts with having enough reasons, because when you have enough reasons the price is easy to pay to drive that change, be it with your fitness or finances.

As I began to make more money I saw a pattern occurring. I wasn't saving as much as I thought I could be. Something wasn't right. I had hit a wall with my financial goals, and I knew it had nothing to do with bringing in more money, at that moment with my career. At the time I was making good money. The more I dove into the self-help books and the courses, the more I learned; and the more I learned the more I began to understand that my issues with money had to do with my money mindset. This confirmed for me that Parkinson's Law equally applied to my finances, "expenses expand in relation to your level of income," unless you keep that in check.

What is your money mindset?

It is how you feel about money. It is what you believe about money. It is how you think having money defines you and indeed how you ultimately relate to that piece of paper.

Your thoughts, feelings and beliefs about money can seriously limit your ability to achieve your financial goals. I am more pragmatic than I am woo, and I have experienced a huge shift in how I relate to money, all because of my mindset. This huge shift has had a tremendous impact on my financial fitness.

I am no longer in debt. I have savings. And most importantly, I have a healthy relationship with money. Prior to beginning my mindset work, I did not have a healthy relationship with money. Deep down, from a very young age, I had this erroneous belief that money was the root of all evil. I thought that rich people were bad, and that poor people didn't have money because all of the rich people were holding onto it. I was also made to believe the narrative that money didn't grow on trees, and you had to work hard for it, and this is why I worked so hard!

In order for me to achieve my financial goals I had to retrain my brain to understand and develop a healthy relationship with money:

1. I didn't have to work 100 hours a week to earn good money.

2. Money is not evil or bad in itself, but rather a tool. However, what is dangerous is the love of money that is self-consuming.

3. Rich people aren't bad.

4. Money allows you to do good in the world.

5. Money is the means but not an end.

6. I earn money to be financially free in order to provide for my family.

7. Money is a tool to sustain my livelihood and that of others.

How did I do that?

The first thing I learned and had to come to accept was that being great with money is 80% mindset and 20% knowledge. Yes, you read that right! You can have all of the best tips and tricks for investing and making money, but you will always hit a financial ceiling if your money mindset is terrible.

What is your big reason or why you want more money?

For example, my reason was so I can just have enough to sustain my family and not worry about money. In other words my big *why* is to provide security for my family, and that is the *why* that gets me out of bed earlier every morning, even if I don't feel like it to put in that workout and work on myself. I show up day in day out for my family, for my friends, as a coach, business partner and consultant.

The second thing I did was rewrite my money story. Every single human being has a money story. It begins long before you even say the word money or know how to use it. You watch your parents struggle to pay their bills. Or the holiday movie your family watched every years tells the tale of a mean old rich man who treats people terribly and needs to be taught a lesson about kindness. Whatever your money story is, own it and then change it.

Having money isn't about how much you earn, it's about what you do with the money you earn. As you begin to rewrite your own money story, here are a few affirmations to get you started:

1. Money is a good tool that I can use to do so much good. The more I recognize all of the good it does in my life and that of others, the more it wants to hang out with me.

2. Money is not good or bad. I choose to do good with the money I have.

3. I commit to save a minimum of 10% of my income.

4. I commit to give 10% of my income to people less fortunate.

5. The more money I'm blessed with, the greater impact I can have on the world.

6. It's possible to grow money from anywhere.

You can either read these affirmations to yourself, write them out, or speak them out. Whatever works best for you!

## Simple Recap

This chapter was action packed! There is a lot of great information I want to share with you in this book and so I do want to move on, but that doesn't mean you have to do these exercises once and then never look at them again. I revisit my *why* all the time! I do it when I'm stuck in any aspect of my life. I also regularly do the Look Back

Exercise, and the visualization of a day in the life of the version of me who has achieved his next set of goals.

I want to leave this section with a quick recap of the big picture process. Fold down the page and come back here whenever you are feeling a bit lost:

1.  **Get real with yourself and accept where you are at.**

2.  **Allow yourself to truly feel the pain you want to deal.**

3.  **Get to the root of your really BIG why. If your reasons aren't strong enough you won't succeed.**

4.  **Know where you want to go.**

5.  **Let your *why* guide you to create a mindset for success.**

Chapter 4

___

# YOUR RESOLVE

**"There is no chance, no destiny, no fate, that can
circumvent or hinder or control the firm resolve
of a determined soul."
—Ella Wheeler Wilcox**

When you are determined to change your life for the better, it is your resolve that will keep that determination strong and focused. In this chapter I am going to share with you what I call the 4 Cs, and why they are so important. These four short words are huge! They will help you push through the lows you will inevitably experience as you shift into the higher version of yourself.

What are the 4 Cs?

1. **Commitment**
2. **Challenges**
3. **Coaching**
4. **Changes**

## The Powerful Tenacity Pathway

Before I dive deeper into what these 4 Cs mean to you and your journey, I want to tell you about a concept that forever changed my life. It is called the Powerful Tenacity Pathway. The idea is that once I truly commit to my goals and employ the 4 Cs in my process, I enter the Powerful Tenacity Pathway. This is your pathway to success! Once you are on this pathway, you have given yourself the tools you need to remain tenacious throughout your transformation and beyond.

Once on the Powerful Tenacity Pathway, you will find a way to jump over any hurdle, slow down to manage the speed bumps as needed, and face any challenge with courage and strength.

What is tenacity?

The dictionary definition of tenacity is:

**the quality or fact of being able to grip
something firmly; grip.**

What is resolve?

The dictionary definition of resolve is:

**firm determination to do something.**

When you resolve to achieve something, your tenacity gives you the strength to hold on. Your commitment to yourself and your goals will help you to choose the right support (coaching), to help you navigate the challenges and ultimately accept the changes you need to make to achieve your goals. Once you fully embrace the 4 Cs in your process you will have officially embarked on the Powerful Tenacity Pathway. And let me tell you, once you are on this path you will feel the pull to succeed. You will have entered into the next phase of your development, and even though some days you might feel like it would be easier to turn back, your resolve won't let you.

Your resolve will keep you on your Powerful Tenacity Pathway. Let's walk together through the 4 Cs and get you started!

## Commitment

**"There's a difference between interest and commitment. When you're interested in doing something, you do it only when circumstance permit. When you're committed to something, you accept no excuses, only results."**

**—Art Turock**

In order to be tenacious, you have to commit. There is no way around it. You have to fully commit, both consciously and subconsciously. With every tiny cell in your whole genetic makeup you need to decide to stay the course no matter what is thrown your way.

What does this really mean? How can you tell when you're committed? For me it means that you're not doing it just for the sake of doing it. Think of goals such as marriage. When people commit to each other they make a vow to be with each other through thick or thin, until death do they part. Sure, marriages do end, but most often couples give it a good fighting chance before calling it quits.

Commit to your goal as if you are marrying it! Try out this this fun exercise:

Write vows to your goals. For example, if your goal is to pay off your debt and increase your investments, you could write something like this:

*Money, I've known you all my life. I know all the good things you can do. I commit to learn more about how I can use you as a tool to do good in my life and the lives of others.*

*I choose to spend my money wisely by committing to enjoy the challenge of saving more money to make my dreams a reality.*

*I commit to being disciplined in making hard financial choices now, so I can enjoy an easy life later when I'm in control of my expenses.*

*I'm committed to eliminating all my debts that don't serve me well because I'm ultimately in control of my money and debt does not control me.*

Do you see what I did there? If not, let me give you a few clues. When people have a poor relationship with money it is often because of their own limiting beliefs, some of which might include:

Money is evil. This is a big one! One that often causes people to subconsciously get rid of money as soon as they have it.

Wanting money makes me a bad person. Another common one! This limiting belief may be one that will inspire you to subconsciously block yourself from receiving money in your life.

I took these two limiting beliefs and turned them around to write my vows about how I relate to money. Ultimately I chose to write these vows because it is in making the commitment to understand and appreciate the fact that money is a tool and can do a lot of good that I ultimately allow myself to break free from a cycle of debt and worry.

Try it. What is your goal? What are you committing to? Write some vows to that commitment. If you're still struggling to figure out exactly what to marry, here are a few more examples:

If your goal is to lose weight and become more physically fit, you are marrying and writing vows to your healthy body.

If your goal is to be more present in your life, you are marrying and writing vows to yourself, the version of you that is reading these words in this very moment.

If your goal is to sort out your finances, then write a vow to commit even as little as 30 minutes a week to look at your finances or read a finance book or article.

## Challenges

**"All the energy in the universe is evenly present in all places at the same time. We don't get energy, we release energy. And the triggering mechanism to release energy is desire. When you have a strong desire to do something, you will always have the energy to do it."**

**—Bob Proctor**

Did you read that quote by Bob Proctor? And when I ask that I mean, did you really read it? What Mr. Proctor is saying here is that when you have a goal and your resolve is strong enough, you will always have the drive you need to face any challenge that comes your way.

Another really great quote about facing challenges comes from Zig Ziglar:

**"You can't climb a smooth mountain."**

There have to be ridges. There have to be things to grab onto. If it were smooth you'd never make your way up at all. Why do you need to face challenges in your journey to success? I think that many people may have a different answer for this one, but for me it's pretty simple:

The challenges we face remind us why we are doing what we are doing in the first place.

The challenges we face help us grow stronger in our resolve.

The challenges we face make it easier to get through anything the future throws our way.

Facing challenges is an integral part of your journey. If it were easy, you probably wouldn't commit. If it were easy, everyone would do it. Some of the greatest accomplishments experienced by humans on this earth were done in some of the harshest of circumstances. It is human nature to fight harder when there is a fight to be had, especially when you are fighting for something you believe strongly in.

The big thing to remember is that sometimes you'll fail when you face these challenges. These aren't the times to give up. Failure makes you stronger. Get back up. Backtrack if you need to, but keep going. Get back up and take a breath if you need to, but keep going. Whatever you do, don't stop! It is okay to fail. In fact, I highly recommend it. When you fail, it tests you like no other challenge can. It tests your resolve, it tests your WHY. So fail and keep on failing until you stop failing.

Have you ever met anyone who has tried to quit smoking and has failed again and again and again, before finally kicking the habit? Quitting a habit that is a part of your daily routine is hard. Quitting a habit that is also a physical addiction can sometimes feel impossible. But once you're through it, and know for sure that you will never ever light another cigarette, it becomes worth it. But imagine on that first failure, or that second or third failure, that you decided that you could never do it and so you just gave up? You'd never know what it felt like to be the healthier version of yourself. You'd still feel guilty when you thought about what you were doing to your body. You'd still worry that you were going to be the one to cause your own death. But because you decided to keep trying, even after the fourth failure, you succeeded in becoming the healthier version of yourself.

Do you see what I'm saying here? Keeping with the smoking example for a moment, say you quit for a month and then you have one bad day at work and ask a colleague for a cigarette. You smoke it in the moment and it feels good, but then you immediately feel bad. You've failed. You have a choice here: ether give up completely and go buy your next pack, or give yourself a break, lean into your resolve, remember your *why* and try again. The same goes for your workout. So you miss a day. Sure, it's not great, but it's not the end of the world. Get up the next day and get back on track.

Challenges and failures will happen. These are simply a part of life. Ride the wave and go with the flow. Cut yourself some slack . . . but not too much slack! Get back up and face your challenges head on!

## Coaching

**"There is no more profitable investment than investing in yourself. It is the best investment you can make; you can never go wrong with it. It is the true way to improve yourself to be the best version of you and lets you be able to best serve those around you."**

**—Roy T. Bennett**

One of the best tools you can add to your success kit is someone who will push you to succeed. They will be there when you fall, and when you make it to the top of the mountain. They will be there through all of it to keep you in integrity with your *why*, even if that *why* changes as you grow. They will be the one to give you feedback when you need it. They will be the one to listen and ask the right questions. They will be the one to share the knowledge you need, or to point you in the right direction.

Different coaches do different things. Life coaches often listen to learn and lead in a way that guides you to lead yourself down your own path. Fitness coaches and financial coaches do the same, but they also share some of the knowledge they've learned over the years to help you succeed. For example, as a trainer I can show you how to do an effective squat; one that will help your body rather than injure it. I can also use what I've learned about the body to ensure your workouts are not only safe but equally efficient for you.

Coaches are also great at keeping you accountable. When you are only accountable to yourself, it's easy to succumb to the many excuses your brain might throw your way:

*"Take a break today. You're tired. It's okay. I know you took a break yesterday too, but maybe you can start fresh next week."*

*"Wouldn't it be great if you could get into the office a half an hour earlier and get a leg up on the emails before everyone gets in today? It would feel so good to be ahead of the game."*

*"It's been such a tough week, I know you stopped for a burger last night because you didn't have time to cook, but it's Friday. You deserve to sit on the couch with a cheesy pizza and enjoy a few beers."*

*"You've been doing so well with your savings. I know you don't need to go shopping, but wouldn't it make you feel good? There's tons of room on that Visa, and you'll pay it off next week anyway."*

Excuses. Excuses. Excuses! Your old patterns and ways of being in the world are so easy to fall back into. And once you allow yourself to listen to your excuses consistently, it's harder to get back to your new ways of being. That is when you need an accountability partner. Coaches do that!

But if you're not ready to sign on with a coach or you just don't have the room in your budget right now, I get it. Don't wait though. Just start. Find an accountability buddy. It could be a friend, a colleague or someone you know from the gym. Whoever it is has to make sure to keep you on track. If they aren't calling you out on your excuses, then they aren't the accountability partner you need. In the same way, if you are someone else's accountability partner, listen to them but don't go easy on them. Be the accountability partner they need!

If you don't believe me, lean into the research. It has been proven that you are 92% more likely to succeed in changing your life when you employ an accountability partner. You are that much more likely to succeed when you have someone to answer to. Think about it this way: when you have an idea in your head it sounds amazing, right? You get excited, you feel that adrenaline rush. But then you share your idea with a colleague, and as you're speaking your thoughts out loud you realize it doesn't sound as good as it did in your head. It's the same with excuses. They sound great in your head, but once you have to tell someone why you didn't do the thing you had promised yourself you would do, it doesn't sound as good.

Get an accountability partner! Find someone you respect, who will take your goals seriously. Find someone you can depend on to call you out when you're giving in to your old habits. I can't stress this enough. This one tool that will greatly increase your odds of achieving success, especially in the beginning.

## Changes

**"If you always do what you've always done, you'll always get what you've always got."**

**—Henry Ford**

The 4th C! When you are going through all of the phases, from your initial commitment to facing the challenges to employing an accountability partner to help you through the rough days, the most important thing you can do is embrace the changes.

I know that when you first embark on your journey, you imagine what it's going to feel like when you're healthier, when you're fitter, when you don't worry about your mounting debt every single moment of every day. It'll feel good. You're tired of being in pain. You're tired of feeling tired. You tired of the stress. You know there is a better way to live and you've imagined yourself there.

Imagining yourself there and actually experiencing the transformation are two very different feelings. First of all, your goal isn't really a destination, it's an ongoing journey. For example, maintaining good physical fitness doesn't stop once you are fit; it takes work to maintain your gains. It's a lifestyle change. In order to remain successful, you need to embrace those changes. You have to accept change.

Patterns are repeated in your life because, while you may not like it, the choice to remain in it is comfortable and easy. It's easy to pick up fast food on the way home from work because you stayed late at the office and are tired, because that's what you know. That's what you've done for years, and it's one of the comfortable habits that has contributed to the state of your health now. Change requires work. There is a reason you'll hear many coaches saying, "Get comfortable being uncomfortable!"

To fully embrace change and keep going once things feel a lot less rosy than you imagined they would, you do in fact have to get comfortable being uncomfortable. Think about it this way: when we introduce a new workout, our body aches. For a muscle to grow, it has to experience the discomfort. In the same way, for you to grow, you have to experience some discomfort too.

## Case Study

To give you an idea of how these pillars play into an actual real-life scenario, I want to share with you the story of one of my clients. I have changed her name and some of the details for privacy.

*Michaela originally came to me as a referral from a friend because she wanted a fitness coach. Since having her second child three years earlier, she had found she was so busy balancing work and caring for her children that she didn't have time to care for herself.*

*"Hi Ritchie, it's so nice to meet you. I'm so glad I've finally decided to get started."*

*"Me too Michaela! I want to start today by getting to know you and your goals, so that I can develop an effective plan. Can you tell me what your goals are?"*

*Michaela laughed, "I have so many!"*

*"Okay, let's start with your fitness goals."*

*"Yes, that's a great place to start. I think my biggest struggle right now is my weight. In the last year I've gained at least 20 pounds . . . I think . . . and I just can't seem to take it off. I know I could eat better, but I don't feel like I eat that terribly. So I thought I's start by getting more active."*

*"Great! You are on the right track. Moving your body does wonders for your health, confidence, and will certainly help you take off some of the extra fat. I am a firm believer in short, daily workouts that are effective and fit into your schedule. Before we get started I have a couple more questions for you."*

*"Okay."*

*"The first is: Are you ready to commit to a daily 20 minute routine?"*

*"Yes."*

*"Are you sure?"*

*"Absolutely."*

*"Why?"*

*"Because I want to feel healthy."*

*"Why?"*

*Michaela sat there and stared at me, "Ummmm . . . because I want to feel geed about myself."*

*"Why?"*

*Michaela was getting visibly frustrated, "Ummm . . ."*

*"It's okay. I want you to go home and think about why you want to do this. And I mean go deep and get really intentional. Because there will be tough days. There will be days when it's easier to not bother, and you need to know what is driving you to succeed."*

*Michaela went home that night and came back to me with one of the longest lists I think I've ever seen. She was ready! We worked together for three months and she was feeling great, but there was something else she wanted to work on.*

*"Ritchie, I am so grateful for the work we've done together so far. I wanted to talk to you about another goal I have."*

*"Absolutely."*

*Michaela looked sheepishly down at her hands, "I've been in really bad debt for a long time. I try to save, I really do . . . I just . . . shopping makes me feel good. And now that I haven't been turning to food, I find I am shopping a lot more to lift myself up on the down days."*

*I sent Michaela home again to figure out her why. Here is the list she came back with at our next session:*

*My reasons for wanting to curb my shopping addiction and cut my debt:*

**I worry about money every single moment of every single day.**
**I want to be able to retire when I'm 55.**
**I want to be able to pay for my children to go to college.**
**I want to take control of my life.**

*Short and simple, but big.*

*"Are you ready?"*

*"Yes."*

*It turns out that she wasn't as ready as she thought. We spent hours going through her budget and creating one for her that was reasonable. By reasonable, I mean that we still allotted some of her budget to enjoy some of the shopping that she loved.*

*It was a good plan. But I noticed that with each session, she began to get very vague about her progress with paying down her debt and instead pushed me to just focus on her fitness. The thing that Michaela may have forgotten was that as her coach and accountability partner I wasn't going to let her just drop it without a fight. I knew she had just dropped her budget. This one was going to be a hard one for her. I realized in this case we needed to get to the root of why she was finding it so hard.*

*Without saying anything to her at first I sent her home with a different kind of homework this time. I wanted her to get even stronger in her resolve. The questions I asked her to write on were:*

**What do I believe about money that is stopping me from having savings?**

**Have I attached some of my self-worth to the things I buy with my money?**

*The next time we met, Michaela and I talked about what she had discovered. It turns out that she felt like if she had money then she was taking it from others, but also, that she felt like people only loved her when she was buying them things. So, while we added a small bit in the budget for shopping, she still eat going over in her gift buying.*

*What Michaela ultimately did in the end in order to create a strong resolve, one that would lead her down her own powerful tenacity pathway, was to address her limiting beliefs around love and money. We worked together to strengthen her mindset so that she could commit to facing challenges head on and accept the changes she was making in her life.*

*Michaela's desire to get control of her finances stemmed from the growth she had experienced in her own physical fitness. By taking the time and putting in the energy to get healthy, she was showing herself more love than she had in years. As she did this she realized that allowing herself to believe she had to buy the love of others was taking away from the love she held for herself.*

*In the end, Michaela continues to work with me on both of her physical and financial health, and I am happy to report that she continues to face her challenges with courage, and has succeeded in paying down her debt, shifting her money mindset, losing weight, and loving herself.*

## Self-Reflection

To end this chapter take a moment and answer these questions:

1.  What goal am I committing to today?

2.  What resources do I need to help me face the challenges I will inevitably face?

3.  Who will I ask to be my accountability partner?

4.  What changes to my daily habits do I need to accept?

# Chapter 5

# YOUR REGIME

*"Depending on what they are,
our habits will either make us or break us.
We become what we repeatedly do."*
**—Sean Covey**

Take a moment right now and think about your regular routine. What do you do every single day? What do you put in your body? How do you provide yourself with the tools you need to grow into the version of yourself you know you can be? How are you actively creating the lifestyle you are currently living? Because, make no mistake, you are at the wheel. You get to create the life you want. You get to choose. And it is in your everyday actions that you choose.

It is when you craft your days with intention that you begin to truly take control of your life. This is key: craft your days with intention and watch your life shift in incredibly impactful ways. I know that this shift takes time and work, on many levels. Sometimes you may not even recognize that a habit or action is hindering your progress right away. That's okay. Take the time you need to uncover all of the daily activities/habits that need to either be modified or removed, to help you achieve your long-term goals. On the tough days when you want to slip back into either poor eating habits, work habits or spending habits to feel the familiarity and ease of your usual choices, lean into your new regime to help you through.

So, what exactly does regime mean in this context?

According to merriam-webster.com:

1.  a regular pattern of occurrence or action

2.  the characteristic behavior or orderly procedure of a natural phenomenon or process

To make the big life-changing shifts you know you're ready for now, you need a regime. The key to succeeding with your fitness goals especially is a regular pattern of actions that continuously lead you towards, not away from, your goals. When you repeat an action again and again and again, it becomes a characteristic behavior. You establish a process, it may feel unnatural at first, but with repetition and time it will feel natural.

In all honesty what I am about to share with you in this chapter could be the topic for an entire book. That said, this book wouldn't be complete if I didn't address it at all. If you find you're craving more on this topic, head on over to my website, **www. bodyandbankconnection.com,** or email me directly, **support@ mybodyvitality.com.** So keep in mind as you read this chapter that I'm writing more from the macro; there is a micro element that is too important to try to fit into one chapter. So please don't take the knowledge that I'm sharing here and attempt to apply it to your life exactly as it is. You'll understand why as you continue on your journey.

## The Practical Fuel Formula

**"We all know that humans cannot live without food. Your body is made of the food you eat, and therefore neglecting to consider what and how you eat is the same as neglecting your body. By neglecting your body you are neglecting your mind."**

**—Shoukei Matsumoto**

I help each of my clients to develop a way of eating that will see them achieving their own personal peak performance. Human beings are not like cars at all when it comes to fuel. There is no one-size-fits-all. Following someone else's model of eating, even if they swear by it, will not give you what you need to achieve your best, because your needs are unlike anyone else's. I'm not just saying that to make you feel good. Your body is in fact very unique.

The necessary fundamentals that you need, physically, mentally and spiritually, while similar to others, are unlike those of anyone else on this planet. Each and every one of us has our own threshold for pain, stress, financial burden, worry, and grief. You manage your stress both physically and emotionally in a different way than I do. I manage my anxiety differently than the guy who was standing behind me at the grocery store yesterday, and he manages it differently than the lady working out next to him in the gym today.

Although as humans, we may seem the same in many ways, there are slight differences that make you, you, and me, me. These differences need to be addressed in the fuel we feed our bodies. For this chapter I am going to focus on your nutrition, although I recognize that fuel for peak performance involves so much more than that. Like I said earlier, if you want to chat more about this topic, you know where to reach me!

## You Are a Ferrari

Okay, okay . . . I know I just said that the fuel you need as a human is nothing like the fuel you use in your car. That is true, because you can't just pull your body up to a gas station, quickly spend a few bucks, and off you go. That said, if you were to compare your body to a car, make sure it is a Ferrari. You are a highly complex machine that deserves the premium fuel.

Physical health is 80% nutrition and 20% exercise. Let that sink in!

To demonstrate what I mean I'd like to share a quick story with you:

### <u>A Tale of Two Clients</u>

### *Meet Emma*

*It was Tuesday evening at 7pm when I first met Emma. I remember it had rained unexpectedly that day and she had been caught waiting under an awning at a shop just around the corner.*

*"I'm so sorry I'm late. I didn't have an umbrella with me and I got stuck."*

*"No problem at all Emma. It's so nice to meet you."*

*She smiled but still seemed flustered as she sat down across from me.*

*"I'm never late. Really. I promise this won't happen again."*

*"It's not even 5 minutes. Don't worry at all. Why don't we just get started?"*

*"Sure."*

*"Tell me a bit about why you'd like to hire a trainer."*

*"Well . . . I really am not 100% sure yet. I came today to see if you could help me figure out what I'm doing wrong. I'm very active. I take classes every day . . . yoga, pilates, and sometimes spin, although I don't like those as much. I also go for hikes regularly on the weekends and on some mornings I've tried to run although I'm not sure that's right for me; I really feel the impact on my knees. Either way . . . it doesn't matter what I seem to do, I don't lose any weight."*

*"Okay, can you briefly tell me a little bit about what you eat in a day?"*

*"Honestly, I feel like I really don't eat much. I barely snack. I usually eat yogurt and granola with some fruit in the morning, and a normal sized lunch and dinner. I have friends who seem to be able to eat anything and they are still thin. I'm so frustrated! No matter what I do nothing works."*

*I could tell that the way Emma was feeling about her body was greatly affecting the way she felt about herself. As she spoke the last lines she unsuccessfully attempted to keep the tears from falling.*

*"I'm sorry . . . I just. It seems so easy for others. It just . . . it gets to me."*

*"I understand. I struggled with my weight for a long time. It's not about how MUCH you work out, but HOW you work out. It also isn't always about how much you eat, but what you eat and when you eat. You have to do what's right for your body, and it's all about finding your unique balance. Are you ready to give something new a try?"*

*"Absolutely!"*

### Meet Gary

*Gary walked in with a huge smile and some big confidence for his tiny frame. He shook my hand with strength before sitting down.*

*"Ritchie, it's so good to meet you. My friend John highly recommended you, and I'm hoping you can help me too."*

*"Great to meet you Gary! Tell me about your goals."*

*"I've always been on the skinnier side. I've never really worked out or focused on being physically active, but lately I've been feeling really run down. I'm tired all the time, and doing simple tasks like lifting a box up onto a higher shelf feels hard. I feel stiff when I move sometimes and I think I'm way too young for that. Also, I was thinking it might be nice to have some muscle . . . you know . . . maybe bulk up a bit. I've always thought it might be nice to not be the scrawniest person in the room. I dunno. What do you think?"*

*"Really, it's all about you and how you feel. Getting more physically active will help with your energy levels for sure, and will also really help with the stiffness. But also, a lot depends on what you are eating as well. Without the right nutrients, it can be difficult to build muscle."*

*"I see. So how do you work?"*

*"I take an overall look at your nutrition and daily fitness routines. I compare what you are doing with your goals and structure an individualized plan that will help you achieve your goals. I support you throughout the process and regularly evaluate your regime to make sure it is perfect for your needs."*

*"That sounds great. Can we get started right away? I'm so ready to feel better."*

### The Outcomes

*Both of these clients came to me with one common goal: to feel better in their own bodies. That said, their individual challenges and needs differed greatly. If I had given them cookie-cutter plan based on techniques that had worked for someone else, they both would've failed in achieving their goals.*

*For Gary, we adjusted his eating habits to help him build muscle and gain a bit of weight. Prior to seeing me he simply ate what he wanted to when he wanted to. He snacked regularly throughout the day, but very rarely ate big, heavy meals. He had done a great job of keeping his metabolism nice and quick, but for his goals he needed to slow it down a bit. He did this by going back to 3 meals a day, with a larger dinner loaded with good fats and carbs. He cut down on his snacking.*

*I geared his workout to build strength, and focused on helping him gain more muscle mass and strength. One of the outcomes that Gary didn't expect to happen from our work together was becoming more organized in his daily schedule. As he created the routine of eating and working out at approximately the same time each day, he also structured his work around these times. Gary was a freelancer who worked from home. Prior to shifting his health habits, he often worked as he needed to, working all night to meet deadlines, and taking work as he needed it.*

*As he changed to achieve his goals, he realized that he wasn't able to work out if he hadn't slept, which made him feel worse. Also, his erratic work schedule wasn't helping with his eating. When working long hours through the night to meet a last-minute deadline it was hard to take the time to cook a good meal. Gary would fall back into snacking to get through to the end.*

*So, as his eating and work out routines became more consistent, so did his work/life balance. He began working regular hours and scheduling his projects to not have the rushed deadlines. One of the benefits to this was that he could actually take on more work, and began making more money.*

*For Emma, we had to try a few different approaches. At first she didn't mind dropping her classes to have individual workouts with me, but within a few weeks she quickly realized that she enjoyed those classes for other reasons too. She especially loved her yoga classes because they helped her to relax. She had made a lot of friends through the class and so the social aspect was also very healthy for her. We changed her schedule to include both classes and workouts with me.*

*As for her eating habits, Emma began by keeping a journal of everything she ate. It turns out that the way she was eating and the amount she was eating wasn't right for her body. Although it took some convincing at first, and wasn't successful immediately, Emma ultimately achieved her weight loss goals by combining intermittent fasting, a reduced intake of calories, and adding more focused physical activity to her routine.*

So you see: no two people are alike. Even if you identify more with Gary, it doesn't mean your plan will be the same. Your bodies are different, your lifestyles are different, and so your needs are different. If you give your body sub-standard fuel you won't be able to perform at your best. On the other hand, if you give yourself premium fuel you give yourself the opportunity to experience peak performance on a daily basis. When you feel good, you have energy, and when you have energy you can do anything you set your mind to.

## Not All Calories are Created Equal

**"Let food be thy medicine, and let medicine be thy food."**
**—Hippocrates**

To go back to our examples from above, one of the things that was hindering Emma in her weight loss goals was the types of carbs she was eating. If she needed a quick afternoon snack she'd grab a handful or two of potato chips. It wasn't a lot and it served to curb her cravings for the moment, but in the end it only served to make her even more hungry at dinner, causing her caloric intake to increase at that meal.

Gary was doing something similar, by snacking with carbs that are more filler than fuel, causing him to reach for more of the same throughout the day. These snacks served to make him even more tired, which slowed down his productivity, causing him to work longer hours.

Not all calories are created equal! For example, you may feel a quick burst of energy from a Snickers bar, but it won't last and then you'll have to work through the sugar crash. Whereas the calories from an apple provides nutrients and long-lasting energy.

Your body is sophisticated and complex, but it is also incredibly smart. It is not simply a vehicle for the brain. Everything works together. The food you eat not only fuels your physical energy; it also fuels your emotional responses to tough situations as well as your ability to think. Throughout the day your body is regularly communicating what it needs to your brain, and vice versa. When you are hungry, it is your body telling you it needs nutrients.

When you give your body empty food, like a chocolate bar or a bag of chips, it will become hungrier sooner. There wasn't enough nutrients in the food you provided to fulfill your body's needs. The first thing you can do to ensure success is to give yourself some super helpful tools. For the remainder of this chapter I would like to share a few of my tools with you.

## Get a Personalized Nutrition Plan

Yes, I know I may sound biased here and you know what . . . I am! I am a certified nutritionist and I also work with a lot of colleagues who are also very good at what they do. Hiring a professional to help you craft a plan to provide your body with the most suitable fuel for your own peak performance is one the most valuable investments you can make for yourself.

Think about it this way: when you have a problem to solve, and after trying every possible way to find a solution, but you can't, what is one thing you do? Seek the help of an outside source. Why? Because often they are able to see what you are not, being too close to the problem. It's the same with your nutrition. Of course you know your body better than anyone else in this world, but you probably don't have the same knowledge as someone who has devoted years to learning about what feeds the body the best nutrients.

I can't stress this enough: get a personalized plan from a nutritionist. You can't gain the knowledge you need to create one yourself by reading a book or two. Yes, you can continue to live your life as you are, but I promise you that you will not be operating at your highest level. The problem is, most diets out there are not sustainable because they are instruction-based, cookie-cutter solutions. These generally work for very few people, if any at all, as a long-term solution.

What I really want to emphasize is that, as opposed to following instructions or restrictive diets, you need to learn the fundamental nutrition skills that will not only shift that extra body fat around your waistline, but also empower you with nutritional lifestyle skills that you can take with you forever. That is always my goal with my clients: to give each one the skills to maintain a healthy lifestyle long after we complete our work together.

Yes, I do create individualized plans for each of my clients, but ultimately it's to teach them how to change their lifestyles, and how they relate to food, so they are equipped for life and don't have to worry about putting on that extra weight again.

All this said, here is a macro look at nutrient balance to get you thinking about how you are feeding your body. Macronutrients are types of nutrients that your body needs in larger amounts, and we will cover the 3 main ones in the following pages:

1.  Proteins

2.  Carbs

3.  Fats

**A few key points about protein:**

1.  Protein is known to be a building block for muscle tissue.

2.  The more muscle tissue you have, the more calories you are likely to burn.

3.  Protein helps burn more body fat.

4.  Protein is equally for maintenance and repair of bones, connective tissue, hair, skin and hormones just to mention a few.

5.  Although not its primary role, protein is a source of energy. A single gram of protein provides 4kcal of energy.

6.  Protein is the most satiating (filling) macronutrient per gram, which is awesome for fat loss.[8]

**A few key points about carbs:**

1.  Carbs have been given a bad rap when it comes to fat storage, but eliminating carbs altogether can be detrimental to your overall gut health.

---

[8]  https://www.ncbi.nlm.nih.gov/pubmed/17023705/

2. Without carbs (not the sugary, highly processed ones) cortisol levels will be higher.

3. If your carb consumption is right you should not have cravings. It will also help lift your mood and keep your energy up.

4. The main role of carbs is to provide energy.

5. Carbs are what are referred to as non-essential nutrients in relation to the other two (protein & fats), meaning you technically can survive without carbs. Although carbs are not essential to your diet, it is almost impossible to have zero carbs in your life due to amounts of carbs contained in foods such as vegetables and fruit.

6. A single gram of carbohydrate provides 4kcal of energy.

**A few key points about dietary fats:**

1. Again, dietary fats are not the enemy some have made them out to be.

2. Dietary fats are not the same as body fat.

3. Omega 3 and Omega 6 are both key fatty acids which are essential nutrients. Omega 3 in particular is high in DHA which is good for memory and reaction response, among other things.

4. Dietary fats are key in maintenance of brown fat (brown adipose tissue), which is good for cranking up your metabolism as it triggers the burning of white fat.

5. The main role of dietary fat is to provide an energy source.

6. A single gram of dietary fat provides 9Kcal of energy, which is more than double the energy source per gram coming from protein or carbs.

Studies have also found diets higher in dietary fat resulted in improved fat loss results as opposed to diet higher in carbs and lower in fats.

Your overall gut health is more important than you might think in helping you achieve all that you want to in a day. If you are anything like I used to be, food takes a backseat to your work. For me, food was always an afterthought, which led me to barely think about what I was putting in my body at all. I would grab anything on the go to satisfy my hunger, which led to some very poor eating habits.

A huge factor in your weight loss goals being sabotaged is inflammation. Foods that are high in processed sugars or artificial trans fats help to release inflammatory messengers in your body, which over time can lead to chronic inflammation. The best way to fight inflammation is to eat nutrient rich foods and make time to exercise!

When you think about the food you're eating, know that it is always okay to include carbs, proteins and dietary fats, but you have to create a balance that is right for you. Everything in moderation!

## Meal Prep

DO THIS ONE THING AND I GUARANTEE YOU WILL SUCCEED!

I am not kidding. Set yourself up for success by preparing ahead of time. The easiest way to fail at creating healthier eating habits is to not be prepared for those moments when you're really hungry. Sometimes the thought of prepping food for the entire week can seem either overwhelming or boring.

I have a system that is easy, takes very little time, and ensures that the food you have made for yourself is always fresh.

First of all, I don't prep for the entire week at once. I prep meals on Sunday and Wednesday. Begin by choosing 2 days of the week that work best for your schedule.

Think about your food in terms of the three macro nutrients I talked about above:

**Protein** – pick 3 or 4 that you enjoy the most that you can rotate through

**Carbs** – choose 2 to 3 good carbs

**Fats** – this is flexible

On Sunday (or whatever day you choose for day 1), prepare at least 2 proteins and 2 carbs. Portion them out into meals for the next four days. Also portion out some healthy snacks that you can take with you on the go. Peanuts, for example, are a good healthy fat and a great snack.

On Wednesday (or whatever day you choose for day 2), prepare 2 different proteins and 2 carbs as well as your snacks.

If you find you get bored with the food you prepped and you have time one day to make yourself a healthy meal, don't fret! Just put your prepped meal in the freezer and save it for one of those days when you may not have as much prep time as you need.

## Intermittent Fasting

This has worked brilliantly for me and for so many of my clients. It's generally been taught that in order to have a healthy eating routine you must eat breakfast in the morning when you get up, and this is simply not true. The word breakfast quite simply means to break your fast. You can choose to break your fast whenever you like.

The most effective breakdown is 16 hours to 8 hours. What this means is that you are only eating for 8 hours in the day. You begin the eight hours at your first meal and make sure to have your last meal or snack at the end of it.

The one thing to remember is that this is not a diet, it is a lifestyle. There are more benefits to intermittent fasting, and a lot of research to prove them. Head on over to my website for more resources if you'd like to learn more: www.bodyandbankconnection.com

## Food, Health & Your Finances

How does this all apply to money?

First of all, just like your body and your brain and all the cells are interconnected and affect each other, so are the other aspects of your life. When you feel healthy, you have a desire to be the best you can be in all areas of your life. When you have energy, you can think more clearly. You can see where you need continued growth and development. If the heavy weight of your debt or worry over your lack of savings for the future is bringing you down, you'll want to fix it.

But also, saving is connected to weight loss in an even simpler way: it's all about self-regulating. Losing weight and watching what you eat is budgeting. It's a skill you are developing. Budgeting your food intake is like budgeting the flow of money to and from your bank account.

Eat what your body needs for your physical health.

Feed what your budget needs for your financial health.

## Pay Yourself First

The ultimate takeaway from all of the knowledge that I have shared not only in this chapter, but in the first four as well, is that you need to pay yourself first. Nutrition is your ultimate key to success. By feeding your body the right fuel, you help yourself operate at peak performance in all areas of your life. This in turn allows you to be a healthier and happier mother, father, daughter, son, friend, colleague and community member. You lead by example when you pay yourself first!

## Healthy Recipes to Get You Started

**Head over to the book website, www.bodyandbankconnection. com for a sample 7-day meal plan for fat loss and peak performance.**

# Chapter 6

# YOUR ROUTINE

**"Success is the sum of small efforts—
repeated day in and day out."
—Robert Collier**

The quickest, easiest and most effective way to prolong your life is to get fit. It's that simple.

*"But wait Ritchie, it's not that simple at all. I'm busy. I've got three kids under the age of 10, a full-time job, and ailing parents. I don't think I can squeeze anything more in my day."*

*Meet Maria. She has been a stay-at-home mom for the past 7 years, and recently re-entered the workforce. She knew she had to do something for herself and had always wanted to go back to work, not only for herself but for her family.*

*Maria believed that the best way to raise her children was to lead by example. With all of them in school, she knew it was time to get back to work on herself, but the reality of achieving her goals a little later in life was weighing on her. Not to mention all of the pressure she was under being the sandwich generation. It was a lot.*

*I met Maria one day on her lunch break. She had heard about me through a friend and was curious.*

*"Thank you so much for meeting me, Ritchie. I don't think I have time to work with you, but I wanted to . . . well . . . I don't know. I feel like I'm letting myself go physically and as I get older it seems harder for me to keep the weight off. I used to be able to eat anything and everything and never gain any weight. But not anymore. I'm also exhausted all the time. I don't think I remember what it feels like to have energy. Did I ever even have any?"*

*"Of course you did, and you still do. A great thing about what I can do for you is to show you that if you spend 20 minutes a day on a quick and very effective workout, you'll have even more energy than you would if you hadn't. I know it's counterintuitive. You think that you'll be tired after a workout, but you will actually feel invigorated both physically and mentally."*

*"Wow! I feel like that might just be too good to be true."*

*"Ha . . . are you willing to give it a try?"*

*"Yes . . . yes, I am."*

What if I told you the same could be true for you too? You might be thinking that your situation is nothing like Maria's. You might have a job where it's normal to work 12 hour days, or you work shifts. You might be working with injuries or physical limitations. It's okay. Don't let these things get in your way. There is a workout for everyone. It doesn't matter how busy you are, or what other challenges you are facing. My promise to you is that there is always something you can do to get physically fit.

This all starts with having a strong enough reason to look after your health and wellness. This was a concept we covered when we talked about the Dynamic Drive Accelerator. I always tell my clients that if you have a strong enough reason you will always find time to go after your fitness or health goals. Your reason or big WHY will drive you to take action. It may be hard at first, which is why we need that reason to propel us until our actions turn into a routine, which with repetition forms a habit.

## The Proven Metabolic Protocol

One of the things that held me back from getting in shape was the misconception that I had to spend hours at the gym to achieve my fitness goals. Once I learned that this is just not true, and embraced this truth, it opened up a whole new way of thinking for me on so many levels.

The first thing it did was remind me that choosing to put my health first didn't have to be hard. In the same way, achieving my financial goals didn't have to be hard either. It is amazing how one shift can have such an impact.

Yes, allowing that shift to inspire a lasting change in habits takes commitment. Yes, it can be a challenge to stay the course and shift those thought patterns for good. Yes, along the way there will be challenges. But, that doesn't mean it can't be easy.

I call this the Proven Metabolic Protocol, which has been a game changer for myself and hundreds of my busy clients over the years. I work with each client to tailor their workout to their own body and needs. In this chapter I will provide a sample workout that embraces the proven metabolic protocol principles, for you to test out. But I highly recommend developing a routine that is unique and tailored to suit the individual needs of your body.

### So, what is the Proven Metabolic Protocol?

This is based on proven effectiveness in enhancing your metabolism, from research and studies.

In simple terms, they are short workouts, approximately 20 minutes or less, that can be done anywhere. Instead of having to go to the gym, you can simply get up in the morning and work out before you get ready for the rest of your day. No packing a bag. No leaving extra time for travel. No fussing with having to get ready for work in a crowded change room. No worrying about how much time you're wasting on these things that don't need to be done.

Get up.
Work out.
Feel good.
Get energized.

Let this one small change impact your life as a whole!

But don't take it from me alone. Let's take a moment to learn about the science behind this way of working out. Anecdotally, I can share with you all of the ways I personally, as well as my clients, have experienced it working, but I know that being backed by scientific proof is even better. So here we go!

A good example of exercises that use the Proven Metabolic Protocol are High Intensity Interval Training (HIIT), which includes some form of metabolic conditioning; however, metabolic conditioning is much wider than HIIT and not all metabolic conditioning is classified as HIIT. "HIIT is characterized by bursts of intense exercise followed by rest periods to allow the body to recover enough to begin the next high-intensity interval. To have maximum effect, the bursts should be challenging and the rest periods kept to a minimum (i.e. just long enough to allow the body to recover to complete the next set."[9]

There have been many studies that prove the benefits of metabolic conditioning, and why it's so powerful. I have used these to shape

---

[9]  https://nimbusclinics.com/blog/8-benefits-of-high-intensity-interval-training-hiit/

my own program and those of my clients. There are 8 benefits to HIIT, and therefore to my Proven Metabolic Protocol as well:

1.  **It's efficient** – Your workout is designed for you to achieve the maximum results in the least amount of time.

2.  **Your heart is healthier** – During these quick workouts you strengthen your heart.

3.  **Anti-aging** – It helps slow the signs of aging.

4.  **You reap the rewards right away!**

5.  **Helps balance hormones** – Reduces the production of ghrelin, the hunger hormone,

6.  **There are no barriers to achieving your goals** – Not having to depend on machinery you can work out anytime anywhere making it easy!

7.  **Blood-sugar balance** – Studies have shown there are benefits to blood flow and vessel dilation.

8.  **Lose weight, not muscle** – This type of physical activity promotes muscle growth!

But the most valuable benefit to the Proven Metabolic Protocol is improved mental health. Studies have proven time and time again that moving your body increases the happiness hormone serotonin. If you take the time to work out every single day you give yourself an extra hit of joy to help you through some of the more challenging times. Not only that, when you feel better about your body, you feel happier. And when you achieve your goals you feel better about yourself as a whole, which also makes you happier.

If you want to read more, I've shared the links to some interesting abstracts in the references section at the end of the book on the following topics:

The effects of high-intensity interval training on glucose regulation and insulin resistance: a meta-analysis.[10]

Acute high-intensity exercise-induced cognitive enhancement and brain-derived neurotrophic factor in young, healthy adults.[11]

## Being Strong Doesn't Make You Fit

**"Take care of your body. It's the only place you have to live."**
**—Jim Rohn**

There are so many misconceptions around the types of workouts that help our bodies achieve optimal health. You've seen the guys at the gym who build a lot of muscle and can lift an incredibly large amount of weight, but they are still not in shape. The way that they are working out their bodies is not optimal. They are strong but that is all.

Fitness is all about balance and commitment. But as I've said many times before, it doesn't have to take over your life. It can be efficient and effective. Work smart! Your body will thank you. How often in your daily work or home life do you search for efficiencies? Often, right?! The more efficient you are, the more you can accomplish in a day. It is no different with exercise. Keep it easy to achieve and you'll face less challenges.

Here are a few more quick points to help shift your mindset around having the proven metabolic protocol become a daily routine in your life:

### When eating an elephant, take it one bite at a time!

Okay, I know it's a weird metaphor but it works. If you were to look at the size of an elephant, knowing that you had a goal to eat it all

---

[10] https://pubmed.ncbi.nlm.nih.gov/26481101/

[11] http://www.ncbi.nlm.nih.gov/pubmed/27450438

one day, the task at first might seem very overwhelming. Elephants are not small creatures! Losing weight and getting in shape can feel the same way: like a huge, overwhelming task. It doesn't have to be. Think of it in the same way you would approach eating an elephant. Start by taking your first bite, chew, and swallow.

Are you still hungry? Did it taste good? Yes! Great, take another bit and keep repeating. You will get there. All you have to do is that that first bite, which leads me to my next point:

### Just start!

Seriously! In a way, by picking up this book you've already begun the process; you've decided which part of the elephant you are going to eat first. Now it's time to take the first bite. At the end of this chapter I am going to provide a sample workout plan for you to test. If you're ready, flip forward a few pages now and go for it! Don't think about it too much. Don't over-analyze it. JUST START!

### Don't let the excuses creep back in.

You will face challenges. Your 2-year-old will develop a cough and keep you up all night. Your boss will take on an extra client on a rush project and ask you to work late for a few days. You'll feel tired and that little voice in your head will say, "Just take a day off, you deserve it!"

Don't listen. Push through and take another bite. Sure enough, with each bite that elephant will get smaller and smaller, until one day that huge task will feel like nothing at all.

### Don't go from zero to one hundred.

I've seen this happen so often throughout my life, not just with my clients, but also with myself, my family, and my friends. You get excited about achieving a goal when you first decide it is one you're going to work at achieving, and so you dive right in with all you've got. The problem with doing this is that it's not sustainable.

If you want to be successful at achieving your goals, take your time. Integrate the changes in your life in a way you can maintain daily going forward.

### *It's all about the movement.*

*"Disuse Erodes Value"—Ritchie Nkana*

Your body needs to move. Many of us tend to spend the majority of our days sitting for long periods of time, only to move when we need to get from place to place. This just isn't healthy. Your body needs to move. I can say this again and again and again. I will never ever get bored of saying it. YOUR BODY NEEDS TO MOVE.

Exercising isn't so much about the exercises. It's about the movement. Get your body going in a way that ensures you will stay physically active throughout your entire life. Have you heard the saying "if you don't use it you'll lose it"? The less you use your body, especially as you age, the more mobility you lose. It can be harder for your body to recover from injury and illness when it doesn't have any tools to fight with.

### *You always have time.*

With the Proven Metabolic Protocol you always have time in the day to complete your workout. When your mind starts listing off all of the other things you could be doing instead, simply remind yourself that you will be able to get all of those things done even more efficiently than you would have, had you not worked out.

## The Afterburn Effect

I have to say that the Afterburn Effect is one of the perks of this type of physical activity that gets me the most excited. It's the equivalent of automating a process at work or hiring someone to do all of the things you don't want to do. It's the same as making passive income while you sleep. It's amazing!

The Afterburn Effect is essentially when your body continues to burn fat for up to 48 hours after you work out. Yep, it's true! I know it sounds too good to be true, but it's not. The Proven Metabolic Protocol is designed to enhance fat burning even while you sleep. How amazing is that? I personally think it's incredible, especially once I began to feel the changes in my own body.

This awesome phenomenon is called EPOC (Excess Post Exercise Oxygen Consumption) otherwise known as afterburn. This is an increased rate of oxygen intake following a high intensity workout which is accompanied by an elevated consumption of fuel, achieved by the breaking down of fat stores. The increased oxygen consumption post exercise elevates the metabolism or rate at which calories are burned, while the body is being restored to its pre-exercise state.

## Your Proven Financial Protocol

**"The secret of getting ahead is getting started. The secret to getting started is breaking your complex overwhelming tasks into small manageable tasks and then starting on the first one."**

**—Mark Twain**

As always I tie my physical practice to my financial ones. Once you feel the connection you'll understand why. It's all about habits. It's all about discipline. But most importantly:

## IT'S ALL ABOUT EFFICIENCY!

*"But wait Ritchie, it's not that simple!"*

*"Actually, Maria, it really is."*

*"I don't understand. How can I be more efficient with my money? I know for sure that I could budget better and that I could be more frugal, but efficient?"*

"How long have we been working together now, Maria?"

"Hmmmm . . . I think it's been just over two months now."

"And in that time, how much have you achieved?"

Maria's face brightened. "Wo much! I feel amazing and I get so much more time in the day to do all that I want to do. I had no idea that giving up 20 minutes every day would allow me to do so much more."

"Right, and not only that, you've come so much closer to reaching your weight loss goals."

"I have!"

"Do you know why?"

"Okay . . . Ritchie! I get it. I get it. By being efficient in my workouts I've given myself more energy to do other things. I still don't understand how this applies to money."

"How much energy do you spend trying to remember to pay your bills on time?"

"Oh . . . well . . . I keep reminders in my phone but sometimes I get sidetracked and don't get to them on time. I know it's hurt my credit rating, but I think I'm better. I don't know, Ritchie. I'm just terrible with money. It seems to fall through my fingers the minute I get it. I really. I just don't know where to start."

"How did you start when you wanted to become more physically healthy?"

"Urg . . . Ritchie, why do you always answer my questions with a question?"

"Because, Maria. You have all of the answers. I'm here to help you find them within yourself. Sometimes it takes a knowledgeable outside perspective to do exactly that. Sooo . . . ."

"Well, the first thing I did was come to see you on a lunch break."

*"Perfect."*

*"And then what did we do?"*

*"You tortured me . . . haha . . . just joking. You taught me how to work out in a way that worked for both my body and my life."*

*"Yes! So, what you're saying here is that you took one small step at a time. But before you took that first step, how did it feel?"*

*"Overwhelming."*

*"Right. That is exactly how you felt when you started your journey with me. So now, we take the same approach with your finances. We'll begin by taking one small step at a time!"*

*"What will we do first?"*

*"Automate a portion of your income for you to keep off the top, and for your bill payments so that they come out on time every single time."*

*"Wow, that's not what I thought you were going to say at all. I thought we were going to sit down and go through everything and do a huge budget . . ."*

*"Nope. One small bite at a time. That way you will be on top of your bills and you will also be building up your savings, besides you cannot spend what you do not see. Just like we did with your workouts. It doesn't need to be overwhelming. With each action you take, it will become easier and easier to manage."*

## One Bite at a Time

Everything you have learned in this chapter about making your fitness routine an ongoing habit can also be applied to your finances. But the key points to remember are:

## DON'T GO FROM ZERO TO HERO

Remember that you've spent a lifetime developing both your money mindset and your habits surrounding both earning and spending. One of the first things I would advise you do is to begin to think about your money mindset. Ask yourself the following questions:

### Do I have any limiting beliefs about money?

If you haven't worked with the idea of subconscious or even conscious limiting beliefs yet, it can be a weird thing to think about. Some of the most common limiting beliefs about money are:

- If I have a lot of money I am a bad person. Rich people are bad and therefore I am bad.

- I don't deserve to be wealthy.

- Money is evil.

- If making money is my primary goal that makes me a shallow person. What good am I doing for the world?

These types of thoughts will make you take actions, whether consciously or subconsciously, that will ensure you never have a comfortable amount of savings. Some of them can also lead you to accumulating an overwhelming amount of debt.

### What can I do to shift my beliefs about money?

I would begin by doing some reading. A book like the classic, "The Richest Man in Babylon" by George S. Clason is a great start; the money principles in this book are timeless and it's also a quick read to get you start learning how the wealthy and successful think about money. Learn how they approach things like asking for a raise or going for the promotion. Sometimes it is the beliefs you don't even know you have that are stopping you from achieving your career goals, and it is directly linked to how you feel about money.

Some people use daily affirmations to shift their thinking about money. This doesn't work for everyone, but a few simple ways to use affirmations are to write them out repeatedly in a journal and reflect on the ways your brain tries to fight them as you are writing them. Place the affirmation somewhere visible, like on your bathroom mirror or fridge, so that you see it every single day. Or you can set a reminder for twice a day in your phone that will ask you to say these affirmations to yourself.

You can educate yourself like you are doing right now. Take courses on money and investing. Or hire a coach to help you shift your beliefs and subsequently your habits.

**What is the first action I will take towards a healthier relationship with money?**

Remember it is just one bite-size step. The easiest one to try first is to take one bill payment and automate it, and remember this is only after you have taken a portion of your earnings for you to keep; paying yourself first is key. Have the payment come out of your account on the same day every month, so that it is one thing you don't have to worry about.

The one thing you absolutely should not do first is try to tackle a whole new budget for your life. This will take time and budgets are not for everyone, by automating you remove that element of self-discipline required to work on a budget and actually stick to it. You need to shift your habits, and just like with working out, this will take effort. Your spending habits play a huge role, whether you realize it or not, on many aspects of your life. If you suddenly ask yourself to not eat out twice a week, you are taking a big chunk out of your social life and asking yourself to sacrifice something that gives you so much joy. So wait before you make the big changes or you are destined to fail.

Thing about that big elephant. To be able to eat it all you need to start by taking one bite!

## PEAK PERFORMANCE/EFFICIENCY

Once you've taken that first step and have begun to automate your bill payments. Keep exploring how you can make your money work for you more efficiently. Work smart, not hard . . . just like you do with workouts. Apply the principles of the Proven Metabolic Protocol to your finances so that you can make money while you're burning fat in your sleep.

## IT'S ALL ABOUT FULFILLMENT

Give yourself the tools you need to achieve both your physical and financial goals, and you will begin to see massive shifts in all areas of your life! You will feel happier. You will be able to address challenges more productively. You'll start playing bigger and living life more fully. Your confidence will soar. Yes, this sounds too good to be true. I promise you that it is not. I promise if you adopt these principles and apply them to your life, you will see results!

- Just like exercise routines are not the means to the end, but rather the means to all of the benefits from exercise, this goes for financial discipline too. What you can achieve with your fitness goals you can also achieve with your financial goals.

- You don't just complete one workout and expect to receive all of the benefits. You need to be consistent and include workouts as a part of your routine to see those gains, and the same is true for your finances. Finances require consistent discipline, and over time will not only get easier but the results will be sweeter too. It's always harder to lose that extra weight than it is to maintain a lower weight. In the same way it's harder to pay off debt than it is to maintain a debt-free life.

- Just like making exercise a habit, thereby requiring less effort or will power on your part, making good financial practices a habit will help you not have to put much effort in the future. A couple easy habits are: scheduling some time a week dedicated to your finances, and automating your payments and savings.

## Sample Workout

To end this chapter I want to share with you one workout to get you started. Try this and if you are ready to learn more, head to my website for a sample 30 day workout plan at: **www.bodyandbankconnection.com**

**Are you ready?!**

**VITALITY TOTAL BODY 20 MIN WORKOUT**

Do each exercise in the following circuit for 1 minute with no break. Repeat for a total of 2 times through.

1. Jumping jacks

2. Alternating backward lunges

3. Push-ups (modify if necessary)

4. Squat jumps

5. Dips (use a chair or bench)

6. Alternating front kicks

7. Inchworms

8. Prisoner squats

9. Mountain climber

10. Rest 1 minute

# Chapter 7

# YOUR RECOVERY

**"We humans have lost the wisdom of genuinely
resting and relaxing. We worry too much.
We don't allow our bodies to heal, and we don't
allow our minds and hearts to heal."
—Thich Nhat Hanh**

Have you ever been so excited about achieving a goal that you push and you push and you push yourself? You don't want to stop because it feels so good to have committed to something and to be working towards achieving that goal. And then what happens? More often than not you burn out, or worse yet, hurt yourself.

Your recovery is just as important as your workout. Without time to rejuvenate, your body won't be able to realize the rewards of your work. A huge element of changing your lifestyle is patience. Give your body time to adjust. Give yourself everything you need to succeed. Your journey to both physical and financial fitness depends on your ability to recover.

This aspect is so important, it is one of the things I regularly check in on with all of my clients. I know it may not be what you think of a coach doing. Yes, I am here to push you to achieve your goals. Yes, I will push you to work hard. And yes, I will call you out if you are pushing yourself to burn out. This is not a sprint!

Changing your habits has to include balance.

## SHAPE

SHAPE your life.
SHAPE your body.
SHAPE your physical health.
SHAPE your financial health.
SHAPE your emotional health.
SHAPE your success.

SHAPE!

In this chapter I am going to share with you the Ultimate Restoration Key to getting in SHAPE.

Here are the elements:

1. **S** – Sleep
2. **H** – Hydrate
3. **A** – Air
4. **P** – Period
5. **E** – Energy

Yes, one of the key components to getting into shape in all areas of your life is restoration.

## Sleep

**"Your future depends on your dreams, so go to sleep."**
**—Mesut Barazany**

What happens to your body when you don't get a good night's sleep? You probably don't need me to answer this one, because I'm sure you've felt it many times in your life. Your body feels heavy. Your brain feels slow. Every task, no matter how big or how small, feels like it is sucking the last bits of energy from your entire being. This is why we get anxious when the clock is ticking into the wee hours of morning and our eyes are still wide open.

Sleep is important to all aspects of daily living. If you want to be productive, get some sleep! I've met many people in my life who tell me they don't sleep, that they function perfectly well on 4 to 5 hours. My argument to this is that they could be getting more done in less time if they got the full 8 hours. Matthew Walker, in his book *Why We Sleep,* talks about why people are cheating themselves when they think they are performing optimally on little sleep. He attributes this to studies that have shown that individuals with chronic sleep restriction over the months and years acclimate to impaired performance, lower alertness and reduced energy levels. He further highlights how, based on epidemiological studies of average sleep time, millions of individuals spend years of their life in a sub-optimal state of psychological and physiological functioning, never maximizing their potential of mind or body due to insufficient sleep.

Other than what you actually feel both physically and mentally when you get a healthy amount of sleep, there are also negative and positive impacts you may not be aware of. The negative impact is that a lack of sleep causes unnecessary inflammation in the body, which can lead to chronic joint pain and a whole list of health issues. One of the positive outcomes of getting the recommended amount of sleep is that it aids in fat loss. Yes, you read that right: A good night's sleep can help you lose fat!

When you sleep is when all of the good stuff happens! Your body heals. Your body restores. Your mind relaxes. Your stress levels drop. You gain energy. You give your brain what it needs to cognitively function at a high level. You wake up feeling like you can take on the world! Why? Because with sleep you can truly operate at your most optimal level.

How can you ensure you have a good night's sleep?

The best way to guarantee that you sleep well every single night is to follow the 10-3-2-1 sleep rule. I picked up this model from one of my mentors, Craig Ballantyne. In his book *Perfect Day Formula* he outlines this formula:

**10 hours before bed**—You stop drinking anything with caffeine in it. Of course, this means coffee, but it also means tea and some surgery drinks as well. If you love a cup of hot tea in the evening, try switching to one that naturally doesn't have any caffeine.

**3 hours before bed**—Have your last meal. Yes, this includes all eating including snacks. Many foods can be disruptive to your sleep pattern, such as chocolate which contains caffeine! This can boost your energy, causing you to wake up multiple times throughout the night. Eating certain foods right before bed can also stimulate the production of acid in your stomach and cause heartburn, which will also take away from your sleep. So do yourself a favor and stop eating before bed. One of the other added bonuses is that you won't be needlessly slowing your metabolism.

**2 hours before bed**—Stop working. Seriously, don't even peek at your email. Everything can wait. You will be more productive in the morning if you allow yourself to shut off. Let go of all thoughts about work. Yes, I know this can be difficult. But if you keep stimulating your brain it will stay awake.

**1 hour before bed**—Turn off the TV and all other devices. The blue light will again keep your brain stimulated and awake.

This is the strategy I always share with my clients to start. Sometimes they need a little more help, and so once they've given the 10-3-2-1 strategy a fair shot, I then dive deeper into other ways that can help them have an easier time of falling asleep and staying asleep. A few other things that have worked:

1. Changing the lighting in the room. Is there too much light spilling into the room from external sources? Sometimes a street light is just outside the window, keeping the room too bright and stopping the brain from getting optimal sleep. In this case, black-out curtains might be a good option.

2. For some a warm shower before bed can help. The warmth of the water can relax the body and the brain, making it ready to crawl under the blankets and let go of the worries of the day.

3. Taking magnesium. Magnesium reduces stress and helps you sleep longer. Yes, melatonin can help you fall asleep faster, magnesium gives you more of that full night sleep you need to wake up feeling energized.

The main message: GET SOME SLEEP! I promise that while you might think 4 hours a night works for you, your body will be better off with double that amount. Of course, there is no cookie cutter approach, but over the years I witnessed huge gains in clients who choose to make a full night's sleep a priority. The importance of sleep for peak performance can never be overstated; this would explain why, of all the outrageous records broken and recorded in the *Guinness World Records* books, sleep deprivation has never been considered due to the dangers involved in not sleeping for long periods of time.

## Hydrate

**"Thousands have lived without love, not one without water."**
**—W. H. Auden**

The human body is 60% water. Your heart and brain are 73% water. Your muscles are 79% water. And even your bones are made up of 31% water. That is a lot of water!

Dehydration occurs when the body loses more water than it is taking in. Some of the early signs that you are not drinking enough water and are becoming dehydrated are feeling thirsty, having a dry mouth or even feeling lightheaded. You will begin to pass urine less and when you do it will be a darker color and have a stronger smell. Being dehydrated can cause a myriad of health issues.

**"Research shows that as little as 1 percent dehydration negatively affects your mood, attention, memory and motor coordination."[12]**

Keeping yourself hydrated throughout the day, no matter what you are doing, is essential to not only maintaining good health but also operating at your most optimal level. Did you also know that staying hydrated also helps you burn fat? It's true!

How much water do you need to drink a day to prevent dehydration? There are many differing opinions out there on this one, and as always I recommend listening to your body and doing what is right for you. If you'd like to have a base to start with, the most common recommendation is 8 8oz servings a day, or approximately 2 liters.

---

[12] https://www.sciencealert.com/here-s-what-happens-to-your-body-when-you-re-dehydrated

## Air

**"Breathe deeply, until sweet air extinguishes the burn of fear in your lungs and every breath is a beautiful refusal to become anything less than infinite."**

**—D. Antoinette Foy**

Lungs are the biggest contributor to fat loss. Studies have shown that 84% of fat loss is achieved by way of breathing out carbon dioxide. Fats are broken down by a process known as oxidation, which requires oxygen. So if you want to burn that stubborn belly fat you better make sure you are breathing intentionally!

The benefits of purposefully breathing are many. Not only do you burn fat with each breath, but you can also calm your thoughts, release anxiety, gain more focus, and become more energized. Breath is life. The more intentionally you breathe, the richer your life will be.

If you do not already have a routine where you take the time to focus on your breathing, why not start now? I'd like to help you get started with a few easy ideas. The first is to simply take a few intentional breaths before you get out of bed every single morning. It won't take longer than a few seconds.

Just after you open your eyes take three intentional breaths:

Breathe in through your nose for a count of three.
Breathe out through your mouth for a count of three.
Repeat this three times.

Do this for a month before adding more intentional breath exercises to your day. Remember, it's not a sprint. Take your time; let yourself get used to the changes you are implementing in your day.

The next step is to add more intentional breathing to your routine. Since you are adding a short workout to each day, this is the perfect place to do it. Before you begin moving sit for a moment and close your eyes. Again, follow the instructions from your morning breathing:

Breathe in through your nose for a count of three.
Breathe out through your mouth for a count of three.
Repeat this three times.

Keep doing this each day until you're ready to add more. One of the best ways to really intentionally sit and focus in on your breath is to meditate. Meditation can often be a challenge to master, especially when you are used to being on the go all the time. My best advice to start is to find some guided meditations to listen to, or to give yourself some imagery to pull yourself out of your daily thoughts. Here are a few to get you started:

*Simple breath exercise without imagery.*

Find a comfortable place in your home where you won't be disrupted.
Close your eyes.
Place your hands on your chest.

Breathe in through your nose for a count of three.
Breathe out through your mouth for a count of three.
Repeat this three times.

With each breath imagine the air push against the palms of your hands, filling your chest with oxygen.

Once you've completed those three breaths place your hands on your belly.

Breathe in through your nose for a count of three.
Breathe out through your mouth for a count of three.
Repeat this three times.
With each breath imagine the air push against the palms of your hands, filling your stomach with oxygen.

Once you've completed those three breaths, stretch your arms up high above your head.

Take one last big, deep breath in and as you do stretch your arms up even higher. On the exhale release your arms and bring them back down by your sides.

Open your eyes.

*Simple breath exercise with imagery.*

Find a comfortable place in your home where you won't be disrupted.
Close your eyes.

Imagine yourself sitting in a completely white space. There is nothing around you.
It's like you are in a very well lit room sitting on a white floor with white walls.
This empty space is your canvas, and your breath is the paint. With each breath you exhale into the space, you create the scene of one of your favorite places to be in the world.

Before you start, decide where you want to be. Is it a room in your home? Is it a beach at your favorite destination spot? Is it a seat at a café overlooking a busy street? It doesn't matter where it is, as long as you feel relaxed and happy there.

Breathe in through your nose for a count of three.
Breathe out through your mouth for a count of three.
As you exhale fill in some of the scene.

For example, if your place is a deserted beach in some tropical place, as you exhale that first breath, imagine the sand filling in beneath your body.

Breathe in through your nose for a count of three.
Breathe out through your mouth for a count of three.
As you exhale fill in more of the scene.

For example, in my beach scene I would fill in the calm ocean next. A light tranquil blue would continue out as far as my eyes could see.

Breathe in through your nose for a count of three.
Breathe out through your mouth for a count of three.
As you exhale fill in even more of the scene.

For example, I look up to the sky and fill in a soft sun with a few clouds.

Keep going until you have completely painted the world around you in your mind. Once you are done place your hands on your belly.

Breathe in through your nose for a count of three.
Breathe out through your mouth for a count of three.
Repeat this three times.
With each breath imagine the air push against the palms of your hands, filling your stomach with oxygen.

Once you've completed those three breaths, stretch your arms up high above your head.

Talk one last big, deep breath in and as you do stretch your arms up even higher. On the exhale release your arms and bring them back down by your sides.

Open your eyes.

Breathing deeply and intentionally reminds you not only to take some time away from the stressors of daily life, it also gives both your body and mind some time to heal. I have shared more meditation resources on my website for you to dive deeper into your practice. Visit **www.bodyandbankconnection.com.**

# Period

**"There is more to life than increasing its speed."**
**—Mahatma Gandhi**

The time you take to rest and recover between workouts is key to your success. It is that simple. This period of time is just as important as your workout. When you are resting is when all the good stuff actually happens. This is when your muscles actually grow.

Studies have shown that inflammation is one of the key hindrances to weight loss. A link has been found to exist in subjects that are obese or overweight to chronic inflammation.

Chronic Inflammation is also linked to lack of sufficient sleep and overtraining, which when unchecked promotes insulin resistance. Elevated insulin levels leads to the slowing down of your metabolism of stored body fat.

Not all inflammation is bad, however, as this is required for purposes such as responding to an infection. That said, if the inflammation is not checked and turns chronic, it can wreak havoc on your body and immune system.

When it comes to taking time for yourself between workouts, rest is a key component to avoid overtraining, which can cause issues other than inflammation, such as:

- Sleep Issues

- Appetite reduction

- Elevated cortisol levels

- Fatigue

- Mood disturbances

- Damage to your immune system

A great thing you can also do for yourself is to incorporate some non-intensive "active rest" routines between exercises, which means you are still being active but also inducing recovery time for your body. This recovery time allows you are to perform at your optimum. Great active rest activities which are not intense and combat overtraining and inflammation include:

- Massage (studies have shown massage to lower cortisol levels and enhance production of other neurotransmitters such as serotonin and dopamine)

- Sauna session (Increases blood flow to injured or recovering muscles)

- Stretching

- Walks

- Light relaxing yoga

## Energy

If you want to dominate your day, having energy is key! How do you get the energy you need? You already know, but just in case:

Work out!
Eat well!
Drink enough water!
Breathe!
Rest!

When you give your body everything it needs to thrive, you will inevitably become more productive. Your cognitive functioning will increase. Your ability to navigate life's challenges from an emotionally intelligent place will increase. Your ability to physically move through your daily tasks will be easier than ever before. The efficiency with which you accomplish your goals will increase.

In order to maximize your energy and use it to your advantage, you have to take care of yourself; and a big part of that is taking the time to rest. One of the big accountability areas my clients struggle the most with is managing the stress in their lives. Stress and worry deplete your energy like nothing else in this world.

All of the above restoration keys are the building blocks that will culminate in you having the energy you need to show up in the day and dominate!

## SHAPE YOUR FINANCES

How does all of this apply to your finances? The answer is simple: let it rest!

We've talked about how important it is to pay yourself first. If you've done this and you've invested well, shift from actively receiving to passively receiving income. In a way this is like breathing life into your investments and letting them use the energy you've given them to work for you.

Rest and let the money flow. Yes, this can happen for you, just as it has for so many others, but as I've said before: It takes time! If you start investing now in your long-term financial health, there will be a moment when you can shift from active income generation to passive income generation. Start getting your finances in shape now so they will one day work for you, even while you sleep.

The prior chapters have been a build-up of strategies to get you financially fit, setting you on the right trajectory to achieve financial independence. One of the better definitions of financial independence, which I have adapted from a Jim Rohn quote, is: Financial independence is the capacity to live off the income of your personally invested assets or resources.

Initially you start off by putting in the effort to generate your desired income, with the end goal of shifting your efforts to make money work for you as opposed to you actively working to generate income. We have been talking about paying yourself first over the last few chapters, which is all about the initial effort to actively start building your nest egg so that over time you let the power of compound interest do the work for you with no effort on your part.

One proven passive strategy is investing in a low cost index fund. Every market is measured by an index, which is basically a mathematical representation or average performance of the group of securities being tracked by the index. Once the average of that grouping goes up, the index goes up, and when the underlying average goes down so does the index.

Index funds are an awesome passive investment due to features such as:

- They track any market segment.

- Less volatile due to the nature of an index being in large groupings.

- No stock selection required.

- No cost required for fund managers.

- Ultimately lower cost due to less activity such as buying and selling.

## The Tale of Two Runners

Elis was one of those people who was good at everything. If he put his mind to it, he could do it. One day he decided that he wanted to learn how to draw. He threw himself into the pursuit. Every single night when he got home from work, he completed his evening dinner routine, cleaned up, and then sat down and drew for hours until he felt he had mastered it. The thing is, Elis did master it, and was actually quite good.

Once he realized he had achieved his goal, he needed something new to master. Learning new things excited Elis. He thrived on setting a goal and crushing it. So when the drawing goal had been crushed, he decided it was time to get back in shape. All that sitting around every day hadn't done him too much good. It was time to run!

Elis had never tried running before. In his younger years he'd been an avid cyclist but over the past few years, physical activity hadn't been his top priority. Now, it was time to get moving. Elis threw himself into running like he did everything else. He went out and bought all of the best gear. He ran every single day until running 5k was a breeze.

He kept on going until one day he decided he was going to run a half marathon. This felt like an exciting goal! Elis was focused. He continued to run every single day, until the morning of the big race came.

Running in the same race was Martin. Martin had been running for years but had never thought it was possible to run a marathon. This year, he decided to take on the challenge. He had been working on setting some higher goals for himself, and this was one of them.

Martin had been feeling like he'd played things small in his life, all because of low self-confidence. He wasn't sure what changed in him, but he'd been starting to feel like he could do more. This race was one of his first attempts at pushing himself out of his comfort zone. But Martin knew that if he was going to succeed, he had to do it right.

Martin got a coach to help him build his running stamina. He trained his body to become stronger. He built up his ability to run over time. He incorporated rest and took days off. On the morning of the run, Martin felt good. The usual side of him that worried about failing caused some small worry, but for the most part he felt confident.

Both Elis and Martin finished the marathon that day.

Elis did well, but near the end of the race, his right knee started to give him trouble. The pain that he'd been ignoring for the past few weeks hit him full force. But he would not stop. Elis didn't fail and wouldn't admit defeat. He kept going and finished at a respectful time. That would be the last day Elis would run in his life though. He had completed his goal and moved onto the next thing. The problem was, that the next time he tried to get into shape the injury he sustained in that knee would come back to haunt him, making it much harder for him to come back to a place of good physical health.

Martin also did well. He felt good for the whole run and ran his best time. Martin continued to run and stayed in great physical fitness, even running marathons well into his 70s. He had established a routine that was beneficial to not only his physical fitness but also his mindset. Succeeding at something he never thought he could do caused Martin to push himself even further in other areas of his life. He went on to become a well-known speaker and life coach.

The moral of the story: get in SHAPE! Give your body, your mind and your finances the energy they need to work for you. Breathe life into all you do, and you'll see life working for you, even when you're resting!

## Chapter 8

# YOUR ROADMAP TO FINANCIAL FREEDOM

> **"Money is a terrible master
> but an excellent servant."**
> **—PT Barnum**

**M**oney will work for you, when you let it know who the boss is! When your money controls you, you will always work for your money! This is never optimal. The only way to obtain the financial freedom you desire is to get your money working for you.

The only way to be a good boss is to be a successful leader. Leaders obtain their success by first gaining knowledge. Leaders understand where they stand, what their goals are, and what they need to do to achieve them. Leaders know how to work with their team to inspire them to work effectively and efficiently. In this scenario imagine your money as your team. If you are a good leader your team will be inspired to give you your best work.

In this chapter I am going to help you to become the best leader you can when it comes to your money. You will begin by understanding what your goals are, where you stand, what you need to do to achieve your goals, and how to maintain growth while you flourish.

If you are anything like many of the clients I have worked with, embarking on this journey feels like a daunting task, for some even more so than achieving their fitness goals. If you have led yourself down a path where you are in more debt than you feel you can manage, or you're not making the salary you desire, remember two things:

1.  The amount of money you make is not your self-worth! Read that again if you need to. This world leads us to believe that the more we make, the more successful we are as a human being. This is just not true. Detach your self-worth from your bank account.

2.  Your financial freedom is not dependent on the amount of money you make. Read that again if you need to! It's the truth. Making your money work for you is what it's all about!

Let's begin!

## You Can't Hit a Target You Can't See

**"Clarity in purpose makes the price you pay easy."**
**—Ritchie N**

Have you ever tried to hit a target you can't see? Since most of you probably aren't hunters or archers, let's think about it this way instead: Have you ever had a client or a boss ask you to deliver on a goal, but they can't explain or define exactly what that goal is?

They'll say things like: "I'll know it when I see it" or "That's exactly what I don't want."

How have the projects gone when working for a boss that can't help you? In my experience they are often less efficient. It takes many tries to achieve your goals, if you even achieve them at all.

Sure it's easy to say you want to achieve financial freedom or that you'd like to be debt-free, or that you'd like to not worry about money. But what do those statements mean, exactly? If your money was in fact an employee knocking at your office door asking for direction on how to help you achieve your goals, would you be able to give them a clear answer?

If you want to achieve financial transformation you need to be able to clearly define what your goals are. Not only that, but your goals need to be both smart and realistic. You should have a number in mind. What do I mean by this? It's the amount you need to make each year to comfortably survive. This is a very personal number. I have some clients who are perfectly happy living on 30k a year, whereas some need to bring in 100k or even 250k to feel financially independent.

Once you know your number you can begin to understand what you need to do to get there. It's not much different than your physical fitness, and this is why I believe these two are so closely linked. When you figured out what your fitness goals were, you thought about where your body felt most comfortable. This is again very personal. It's a balance of weight loss, muscle gain, flexibility, and movement.

Your financial goals include understanding how you can invest the money you make to bring in the passive income you need to feel financially independent in the future. It is the long game. So, how exactly do you come up with your number? What is the smart financial goal for you personally? The best way to do this is to know what your starting off point is. You don't have to make this very complicated, and remember you can always change it later. I'd like to share with you a case study showing how I did this with one of my current clients:

## William's Financial Goals

*I met William about 5 years ago. He originally came to me, as many of my clients did at the time, to get in better physical shape. As we worked together, we talked about his life goals. One of the things that came up as we talked was his lack of confidence. Some of it had to do with his physical shape, but it turned out that that was only a small piece of the pie.*

*During one of our sessions we decided to focus on the whole picture. Sometimes the root of what is holding you back isn't exactly what you think. William had hit a wall in his progress with his health goals; we needed to understand what in his life was holding him back.*

*"You know, Ritchie, I felt like I was on such a role with you in the beginning. It felt good and easy. I had more energy in the day. I was losing weight, but honestly the last few weeks have felt really hard. I don't have the same motivation. I don't feel like I'm making the same progress. In fact, for the last few days I actually feel like I'm more tired now than I was before I started working with you."*

*"First of all, William, these little dips are normal. We all have ups and downs. As with everything in life, there are moments when the road is easy and others when it feels like an uphill battle. The people who succeed are the ones who don't give up. But I am wondering if we need to go a little deeper and figure if there is something more behind this feeling you're experiencing. Do you mind if I ask you a few more questions?"*

*"Of course not, Ritchie. I really don't want to give up. I just want that good feeling to come back again."*

*"I completely understand! To begin, I am wondering if something happened. Was there one particular event that you can think back on that caused you to feel the way you're feeling?"*

*William sat for a moment.*

*"You know, I don't think so. At first I thought it was because I fell behind on a project at work. I wanted to blame my new schedule, but it's not that. I think I was just placing unrealistic goals on myself. So no, I can't really think of one thing."*

*"Okay. I thought you might say that after our conversation last week, but I wanted to make sure. Do you remember what we were talking about?"*

*"Yes. It was a great conversation actually. It has gotten me thinking a lot about where I'm at in my life and why I'm not where I want to be."*

*"Good! Can you get a bit more specific?"*

*"Sure. I've been wanting to ask my boss for a raise for a few months now. I normally only receive one a year but I've taken on more responsibility since my colleague left. I've worked a ton of overtime. And I believe I'm doing a good job. I started to question myself and why I've been hesitating, and I've realized that I have a problem with my confidence. I feel like if I go in and ask she's going to bring up all of the things I do wrong. When I play out the conversation in my head, I end up feeling like I don't deserve the raise. From there my thoughts move outwards to my financial goals. I can't seem to hold on to money. I'm in debt. I'll never be able to retire."*

*"How do these thoughts make you feel?"*

*"Like a failure. I hate myself when I think about how much money I could've been making if I'd gone for more promotions or even moved companies. I've always just been so afraid. I also get so angry when I think about how I've managed my money. I put things on credit cards that I don't need."*

*"Do you want to change how you manage your money?"*

*"Honestly it feels like it's too late. I'm in my mid-forties. What can I do now that will make enough of a difference?"*

*"Do you really believe that or is it an excuse?"*

*William flushed. He didn't like the question. I waited for him to respond. The silence was uncomfortable.*

*"It's an excuse," he reluctantly responded.*

*"You're right it is! It's never too late. But just like with your physical fitness you have to want it, and not only that, you have to believe that you can do it."*

*"I do want it."*

*"Good. Do you believe you can do it?"*

*"I don't know."*

*"Are you willing to try?"*

*"Yes."*

*"Good. Let's start really simply for now. How much is your phone bill every month?"*

*"Approximately $100."*

*"That's not bad. When you pay your phone bill every month you are also going to invest $100 into your savings. Your homework before our next session is to figure out how much you spend a month without going into debt. Take that amount and add in a budget for a two vacations a year. Add it all up to get the amount you need to live on per year that makes you feel comfortable and allows you to do and have all of the things that you love."*

*When William came back for our next session he reported that the amount of money he needed to live on per year that allowed him to feel financially independent was 60k. We chatted about his current income and what he hoped to be making.*

*"William, I want you to push yourself to aim for 70k a year in passive income."*

*"That's crazy."*

*"Looking at your expenses versus your income, I believe it to be doable."*

*"Okay. I'll give it a try, Ritchie."*

*Our conversation inspired William to apply for a higher paying job at another firm, which he did get. His confidence soared and he was back on track, both physically and financially!*

### What's your starting point?

Take a break and write out all of your expenses. This should include your mortgage, car payments, as well as money for food, entertainment, clothing, gifts, and vacations. Take your monthly expenditures and add them all up to understand what your yearly outgoing amount is. This is the beginning. It will give you a basic idea for what you need to live comfortably once you've established a nest egg that is working passively for you.

Here is a little sample to help you see what I mean:

**Monthly Income: 3000**

**Monthly Expenses**

Rent/Mortgage – 800
Insurance – 150
Groceries – 400
Cell phone – 80
Entertainment – 272
Car Payment – 150
Miscellaneous/Clothing – 100
Gas – 90
Bank Fees – 18
Gym – 40

Giving (10% of monthly income) – $300

Savings – $100
Investments – $100
Extra Debt Payments – $100

Growth (10% of monthly income)

Kindle Unlimited – 10
Audible – 30
Books – 30
Optimize Me – 15
Self-Development Course – 40
100 Day Challenge – 10
Save for travel – 165

**Total Expenses – 3000**

If this is your budget right now, you are comfortably living off of $35,997 a year. This is your starting point. But when you make your financial goal, you want to factor in things like:

1. The length of time you need to get your investments working for you.

2. Inflation.

3. Your career growth. You will be making more money.

You also want to ask yourself if you are happy living on this amount of money, or if your goal is to create even more wealth for yourself.

## Get Scared

**"Discomfort precedes growth."**

**—Ritchie N**

One last piece of advice I give my clients when coming up with their financial goals is to: GET SCARED. I want you to push yourself. All too often, when I say come up with a realistic financial goal my clients think that means they have to play it safe. They create goals that are well within their means when they could in fact push themselves just a little further.

When you push yourself to the limit of what is realistic, you will work harder to succeed. It's still attainable, it's just not comfortable. So get scared and challenge yourself to set your goal, within a reasonable limit, higher than you may have originally felt comfortable with.

Just like a muscle, using the same weight or repeating the same exercise will result in the body adapting and getting into a comfort zone, which stunts growth. To foster growth you need to get the muscles outside of the comfort zone, and that's where growth resides.

## FACE IT!

**"There are some people who live in a dream world, and there are some who face reality; and then there are those who turn one into the other."**

**—Desiderius Erasmus**

It can be hard to face your own reality. It is even harder to face the fact that it is often your own choices and habits that have gotten you to where you are today. But that doesn't mean you need to beat yourself up. Sure, you can be angry with yourself for letting your debt get so high or for not trying to save when you were younger. Get mad, feel what you need to, and then let it go.

The past is in the past. What matters most is what you do right now. How are you going to change your reality right now? Be present in this moment! The first step is to face the facts. Are you in debt? Do you need to ask for a raise? Is it time to look for another job? Or, maybe it is time to go back to school and upgrade your skills.

## Financial Statements

I used a simple financial statement earlier in this chapter to help you figure out how much you need to live right now. Financial statements are great because they give you clarity. They are simple and easy to work with. It's all about tabulating both your assets and liabilities to figure out your net worth. You take your assets and put them against your liabilities to figure out where you stand right now. Your income, in the long run, is worth nothing without assets.

## Cash Flow

The thing to remember is that it is never too late. You can always change your reality. Face the facts and move forward into a new reality by shifting your habits. One of the things I ask my clients to do is to figure out the realistic flow of cash in their daily life. It is similar to what we did earlier but a little more involved to start. I don't ask my clients to keep a budget because over time it's not something that most people can sustain. But when you're figuring out your current cash flow, it's good to take a few months to understand where you may be over-spending. Are there areas where you could spend less? Is it possible for you to put more into your investments?

Understanding your cash flow helps you see where the gaps are. It also helps you keep tabs, especially when there are spikes in your expenses.

## Understanding Debt

There is good debt and there is bad debt. Yes, you did read that right! Most often people categorize all debt as being bad, which is simply not true. An example of good debt is a mortgage. When you are putting money into your home you are investing in your future!

As you probably already know, credit card debt is bad debt. When you hold onto this type of debt you are paying the bank unnecessarily, which will impact your ability to arrive at your financial destination. It's counterintuitive to keep paying monthly high interest rates, especially when these are eating away at the investments you could be making. Rather than receiving a return of 10%, you are giving it to the bank.

Remember, when you are trying to achieve financial independence it is all about your net worth. Owning a home adds to your net worth, whereas holding onto credit card debt takes away from it.

The time to face your debt is now. Start paying it down and stop paying the bank!

## Make a Plan!

Once you have your financial statement and your cash flow, the plan is key! As the old adage says, fail to plan and you plan to fail. Your financial statement helps you see where you are at. Your cash flow is your day-to-day awareness of where your money is going. With this knowledge in hand you can begin to decrease your liabilities and increase your assets.

Again, your plan should be specific to you. Reaching your financial goals is a personal journey, and your plan should reflect that.

One strategy I teach my clients, which has been very effective in paying down debt in the shortest possible time, is the Snowball Debt Repayment Strategy. This is effective if you owe more than one account. The strategy begins by paying off the smallest debt while paying minimum payments on larger ones. Once the first debt is paid off then you roll over that payment onto the next, and so on and so forth. In theory the amounts available for repayment will grow quickly as you get towards the larger debt, like a snowball rolling downhill.

Below are the steps in the Snowball Debt Re-Payment Strategy:

1. List all debts you owe in ascending order from the smallest balance to the largest.

2. Pay the minimum payment plus some extra cash you can afford towards the smallest debt until it is paid off.

3. Pay the minimum payment on every other debt.

4. Once a debt is paid off, add the old minimum payment (plus any extra amount available) from the first debt to the minimum payment on the second smallest debt, and apply the new sum to repaying the second smallest debt.

5. Repeat until all debts are paid in full.

## Pay Yourself First

*"In the house of the wise are stores of choice food and oil."*
**—Proverbs 21:20**

I've said it before and I'll say it again and again and again: PAY YOURSELF FIRST. What does this mean exactly? Simply it means to invest in three things:

1. Yourself!

2. Your future!

3. Your financial freedom!

How do you do that? Well, when I say *pay yourself first,* I don't mean to go out and buy yourself some new clothes or a fancy new car or whatever it is that you might want but don't necessarily need. Of course, treat yourself to things that you love, but that's not what I'm talking about here. What I'm talking about is paying into your investments, because it is these investments that will begin to work for you, and this is what you want. PASSIVE INCOME!

When you build your investment portfolio you are ultimately paying your future self. This is the income that will generate the nest egg you will be able to live off later. When you do this you are effectively taking your current active income and turning it into future passive income. I love thinking about money in this way!

When you think about investing as paying yourself, it doesn't feel like a chore. It feels more like a gift. Who doesn't like gifts? The more you give yourself now, the more you receive later!

## Flourish

**"Someone's sitting in the shade today because someone planted a tree a long time ago."**

**—Warren Buffett**

Today you are planting your own financial freedom tree so that you can sit in its shade tomorrow. When one of my clients has achieved their financial goals, they are flourishing. I believe everyone can achieve this; everyone can flourish. It doesn't matter how much you make, as long as you are paying yourself by making smart investments. Get your investments to work for you.

There are two main enemies to smart investing. I call them the two Es:

1. Emotions

2. Expenses

One of the mistakes I see my clients making all the time is that they attach emotion to their investments. Investments are long-term. The market will go up and the market will go down. Let it play and don't worry. Have faith in the market and stop watching it so much. Letting your emotions get the better of you will diminish your returns in the long run. Let go and relax!

The second mistake you want to avoid making is incurring unnecessary costs when investing. Focus on insuring that the investments you are making are at a low cost. You will want to avoid loans and using credit cards when investing. The cost of using a bank or a fund manager can also eat up some of your profits and 80% of the time those actively managed funds don't beat the market. If you can keep the cost of investing to below 1% you can avoid being set back a couple of years on your financial goals.

One of the best ways to invest is through a simple no load, low-cost index fund. Here is some information on index funds from wikipedia.org:

> An **index fund** (also **index tracker**) is a mutual fund or exchange-traded fund (ETF) designed to follow certain preset rules so that the fund can track a specified basket of underlying investments.

> The main advantage of index funds for investors is they don't require much time to manage as the investors don't have to spend time analyzing various stocks or stock portfolios. Many investors also find it difficult to beat the market because no one has the ability to predict the market on a consistent basis.

> Recent studies, such as one recently conducted by Morningstar, continue to affirm already proven statistics that active managers fail to outperform passive funds, including in periods of volatility such as that triggered by the recent pandemic.[13]

Get your money working for you in the same way as your healthy body is, and you too will flourish!

If you need more information or have any questions, please don't hesitate to email me any time. There is also additional information about the knowledge I shared in this chapter available for you on my website.

---

[13] https://www.morningstar.com/articles/1061438/most-active-funds-have-failed-to-capitalize-on-recent-market-volatility

# Chapter 9

# IT'S ALL CONNECTED

**"The part can never be well
unless the whole is well."
—Plato**

Can you achieve financial fitness without physical fitness?

Of course you can. There is no question. Every single person reading this sentence knows some very wealthy people who have neglected their physical health. You may know them personally. You may know them through a friend of a friend of a friend. Or they may just be a public figure you see on the news. Either way, you've seen proof that you do not have to be physically fit to achieve financial fitness.

That said, for many people living in a physically fit body has helped them to either become financially fit as well, or it has helped them to grow their current wealth to even greater levels. For myself, the discovery of the benefits of becoming healthy and fit were immeasurable. As I talked about in the beginning of the book, this knowledge I share with you comes from my own personal journey.

Remember, money is a tool and not an end goal. The realization that money is just a tool was a game-changer for me. Yes, money is important for the all things it brings, like putting food on the table, and for paying for medical bills, shelter and the clothes on our back. However if the operator (you) of that tool (money) is not firing on all cylinders, your performance will not be your best. This means not showing up as your best version for yourself, your loved ones, clients, friends, and employers. Just like a vehicle; if not serviced regularly, it will not operate at the optimum. It will drive, yes, and be of use, but no doubt the lifespan and performance of that vehicle will be compromised over time.

As a child I was very confused by the way this world works. I'd see people sitting in their offices all day, appearing to do nothing and making so much money, while others seemed to work so hard and made so much less. I didn't understand it at all. But given the choice, I wanted to be the guy making more money.

I learned it was important to have skills that were in high demand to get into those office jobs. Not only that, but to be good at what I did. Anyone can build a trench, but not everyone can be a surgeon. If you're going to be a surgeon you also want the quality of your work to be good; otherwise you won't get much work. Who wants to go to a surgeon who has a poor record of fixing the thing they say they can fix? No one!

Another great example I remember learning from the time in my life when I was deciding what I wanted to do with my career:

*One day in a very busy factory one of the machines that was vital to production broke. Having to shut down, it was losing millions an hour. An expert was called in to fix the machine. He took a moment to assess the issue before taking out his hammer and hitting one spot. The machine instantly jumped back to life.*

*The expert turned to the manager and gave him an invoice for 1 million pounds. He was shocked!*

*"That took you not even five minutes to fix and you only needed one hammer to fix it. How is it possibly worth that much?"*

*"It's not about the hammer or the amount of time it took me to fix your machine."*

*The manager looked confused.*

*"It's about knowing where on the machine to hit."*

Before taking my health back, I was chasing one goal: a career that made me rich! I wanted to be the guy with the hammer. Yes, that's the truth. It was my one priority and I was focused.

I worked a lot. I did whatever it took. And my bank account wasn't in a bad place. What I soon realized was that it was never enough. When I got the promotion and the raise that came with it, I kept looking to the next one. I worked more. I worked harder.

I was unhappy. I was unfulfilled. I was unhealthy. I did little to know physical activity. My energy levels were low. There came a point when I realized I couldn't keep going the way that I had. Something had to change, because if I wasn't happy I didn't understand the point. I knew that the best place to start was with my physical fitness. I needed to get my weight under control. I needed to eat better. Most importantly, I needed to get moving.

The more physically fit I became, the better I felt in all aspects of life. This led me to value my happiness over anything else. I worked less, and do you know what happened? I still got the promotions. I still made the money. I was just more focused. I was more clear on my priorities. Do you know what else happened? My bank account grew, not just because of my career but because of the healthier choices I was making. Getting physically fit inspired me to work on all areas of my life. I learned how to get my money working for me in the way that my body was: effectively, efficiently, and with purpose. The key takeaway is that the road to financial fitness and physical fitness need not be binary; both can be achieved in tandem, which will make that journey much more smoother, efficient and full of vitality.

## The 3 Ds

**"Try not to become a man of success. Rather become a man of value."**

**—Albert Einstein**

As I've grown both personally and professionally, I have learned one very important lesson: if you want to stop chasing success from an economic standpoint you need to understand the importance of the 3 Ds.

**What are the 3 Ds?**

1. Difficulty
2. Demand
3. Delivery

**Why are they important?**

1. **Difficulty**—When developing your skills, make sure that you are difficult to replace. If you're doing something that is easy for anyone to do well, like flip burgers, employers won't care if you leave and therefore won't offer you the best compensation.

2. **Demand**—There needs to be a demand for the skill or service you provide. When you have something that other people need but can't or do not want to do for themselves, you will be in demand all the time.

3. **Delivery**—When you are able to deliver a skill or service really well, you will never have to worry. Employers or clients will come to you. Your service will speak for itself, and the best way to become known for what you do is to be good at it.

What happens when you're not difficult to replace?
You will be replaced.

What happens when your skill is not in demand?
You will not be hired.

What happens when you can't deliver?
You will find it difficult to either get the promotion or find new clients.

Simple answers, but sometimes you need to hear them from someone else. Have you ever had an idea that sounds amazing in your head, but the minute you try to speak it out loud to someone you realize it won't work? It's kinda like that. If you're thinking about pursuing something you are passionate about that will also help you feel fulfilled while growing your bank account, ask yourself if this passion will make you difficult to replace, is in demand, and is something you can deliver on. If the answer is yes to all three then go for it, and make sure you can perform at your best.

The only way a company will work hard to keep you, and pay you well for the services you offer because you deliver quality, is if you are the best version of yourself. When you are the best version of yourself you provide value. Looking at it on an economic value basis, the 3 Ds help you understand how to make your passion, your skills, or the product you provide the answer to someone's problem. Provide a solution, and you will be valuable. Provide that solution better than anyone else and you will become invaluable.

How does this tie into the Body & Bank Connection? The answer is so simple: when you feel better you do better. You not only do better in your career, but in your life. When you're not worried about money, you feel abundant. Abundance attracts more abundance!

## Your Brain on Exercise

We all know that exercise helps brain function, and yet we often sit down at our desks all day and then go home and sit on the couch at night. It's easy to get stuck in an inactive lifestyle, especially when getting bogged down in all of life's day-to-day tasks on top of achieving career goals. But if you push yourself to try, you'll feel how much healthier your brain is.

There is something called the Brain Derived Neurotrophic Factor (BDNF), which is a key molecule related to learning and memory.

"BDNF levels are increased two to three-fold after acute exercise when compared to resting conditions and correlate positively with improvements in cognitive functions in humans."[14]

Studies have shown that the beauty of the release of BDNF is that it actually promotes neurogenesis (formation of new neurones in the brain). So it essentially promotes the growth of new brain cells, no matter how old you are.

What this means is that when you exercise, your brain works more efficiently and with greater ease. You've given it the fuel it needs to complete the tasks you ask of it on a daily basis. Your memory retention is better. You have an easier time solving more complex problems. You are more focused, energized and inspired due to the release of dopamine, the neurotransmitter attributed to motivation.

## A Tale of Two Bank Accounts

*Mike and Bill grew up on the same street, went to the same school and had been best friends their entire lives. They both went on to have successful careers; Bill was an architect and Mike was an accountant. They lived only a few blocks from each other in*

---

[14] https://www.nature.com/articles/s41598-019-40040-8

*a nice neighborhood, in comparable homes. Both had similar ideas about money, with moderate spending habits, mortgages, and some savings. For the most part, they were both doing well. I keep the description of their lives very generic for the purpose of proving a point. Obviously, they each faced their own unique challenges in their personal and professional lives, but we don't need to go into that much detail here.*

*I met Bill first. He was in his mid-thirties and had begun to feel like he needed to be more active. He was heavier than he ever had been in his life. The doctor had said he was dangerously close to having high cholesterol levels. He felt tired all the time.*

*"Ritchie, I'm tired of feeling tired all the time. Can you help me?"*

*"Absolutely!"*

*"Where do we start?"*

*"With commitment. How long have you been thinking of doing this for?"*

*"It feels like years."*

*"Good. Have you ever tried to get in better shape before?"*

*"Yes, but I don't think I gave it a real go. It's like when I was finally ready to quit smoking; I knew I was serious because I sought help. All of the other failed attempts I did on my own, without the use of any aids and the longest I lasted was a month. Now, I haven't smoked in 2 years."*

*"Wow, congratulations! That is an accomplishment!"*

*"What felt different about the time you sought help? I know you said you were ready, but what did that feel like to you?"*

*"In many ways, I felt a lot like I do now. I'm tired of feeling tired, in the same way I was tired of feeling like I was being controlled by my need to smoke. I guess it's the same, I don't feel good about*

*my current habits and I know they need to change. Deep down in my gut I understand that they need to change now."*

*"Great! I'm glad to hear it, Bill. I know I can help. Let's get started by building a workout plan that works for your body and schedule. This may take a bit of trying some out to see what works best for you. Does that sound good?"*

*"It sounds amazing. I want to feel better right NOW. I can't wait to get started."*

*"Remember, you may have to be a little more patient to see some gains. If you think the change is going to happen instantly, you'll get disappointed when it doesn't and this may lead to you giving up."*

*Bill nodded.*

*We met again later that week and began his training. As I suspected he struggled a bit in the beginning when it didn't produce instant results, but he stuck it out. There were days when he wanted to give up, but he didn't. Once I had him on a good routine, we tackled his diet. Again, he went all in in the beginning, and had to take a step back a bit when he got frustrated. Once he got into the habit of eating to feel good, rather than to "do what he should," he began to see more consistent success.*

*Bill experienced a very similar result to mine. When he felt better physically, he was more productive. He provided even more value in his work, and this was reflected in the level of clients he was able to attract to his architectural business. Bill realized that he was happier working less and being able to spend some time on the weekends in nature. He began hiking in the nearby mountains. In the past he normally would've been catching up on work throughout the weekend, leaving only some time for social activities and rest.*

*As he began to make more money, he began to wonder how he could get his money working for him, so that he could start to work even less, and hire more people to do what he didn't want to do.*

*About a year after we started working together, Bill brought his friend Mike in to meet with me.*

*"Nice to meet you, Mike, and great to see you, Bill. How can I help you today?"*

*"I want my friend Mike here to start working with you. He didn't want to come today. I bribed him with the offer of free dinner after!"*

*Mike laughed, "He's right. Bill has been trying to get me here forever, but honestly I don't think it's going to work for me. I don't have time right now. First of all, I don't own my own business, I have a boss, and that boss expects a lot from his top people. I do well because I work hard. Once I get a little further ahead I can stop and focus on other things. But for now, I just don't know."*

*"So then why did you come?"*

*"Free dinner."*

*"Nah, I don't believe that."*

*I waited and looked at Mike. I was doubtful that he would believe me or his friend, but I was willing to give it a shot. This way of living has helped me achieve so much happiness in my life that I can't help but want to share it with others. I know that we are all unique, and so what works for me may not work for others, but if I have the chance to change even one more life, I'll put in the effort.*

*"Okay I'll admit it, I'm curious."*

*"Good! Curiosity is the best place to start. Are you curious enough to sign on to give a month of working out with me a try?"*

*Mike hesitated.*

*"Can you tell me more about what that means?"*

*I took some time to explain to Mike how the schedule worked, and what the workouts were like and why they work. I knew it would help him. I could tell he was struggling. And so to ease him in I offered to take him on for only two sessions a week for a couple of weeks, so that he could give it a try. He agreed, but after the two weeks he didn't continue. He just wasn't ready.*

*Fast forward two years and Mike came to visit me again. This time he came on his own without any bribing from Bill.*

*"Nice to see you Mike."*

*"Hey Ritchie. I'm sorry I bailed on you the last time, I was just so focused. I couldn't see beyond my work."*

*"Don't apologize. What's changed now?"*

*"I have a family. So you'd think I'd be even busier, and I am, but I need more balance. I also need to plan for the future. I feel like I'm going to burn out if I keep going the way that I'm going."*

*I knew there was more and so I kept chatting with Mike to see if I could pull it out. What he shared with me wasn't necessarily a surprise. I'd felt it and witnessed it in many of my clients. Mike shared that both he and Bill were pretty much on the same level with their earnings, and up until the last few years he knew that they had been reaching the same level in their savings for retirement. But recently Bill had far surpassed him, was working way less, and was so much happier. Mike was ready to achieve that quality of life for himself. He was still focused on achieving success in his career, but he also wanted to have more time with his wife and newborn son, without sacrificing their financial future. He was ready!*

What can we learn from Bill and Mike?

First of all, you can achieve financial freedom without physical fitness. Without having his friend Mike to inspire him, Bill probably would've done fine financially, providing for his family and their retirement.

Second, if you learn how to get your body and your money working for you, rather than working for them, you make the journey that much sweeter. When you are operating at peak performance, you have the momentum to move forward. It's easy.

Finally, we are not just talking about bank accounts! There are so many accounts in your life that provide your life with wealth. Fill your love account. Fill your joy account. Fill your experience account. Fill your fulfillment account!

## Exercise Break!

Take a moment and to reflect on the following questions. If you don't like writing in a journal, that's okay. Simply find a quiet place and think about the following:

1. If I were to start working on my physical fitness today, where would I be in a year?

2. If I were to start working on my physical fitness today, where would I be in 2 years?

3. If I were to start working on my physical fitness today, where would I be in 5 years?

4. If I were to start working on my financial fitness today, where would I be in a year?

5. If I were to start working on my financial fitness today, where would I be in 2 years?

6.  If I were to start working on my financial fitness today, where would I be in 5 years?

7.  If I were to started making my happiness a priority today, how good would I feel tomorrow?

8.  If I valued my life enough, what would I do to live it in the best possible way?

Come back to these questions again in a week, and then two weeks and then three. Put a reminder in your phone. Keep reflecting. Keep growing. Allow your answers to inform your decisions. Growth is a process. Your answers will change as you grow.

## Make Your Journey So Much Sweeter

**"Life isn't about finding yourself. Life is about creating yourself."**

**—George Bernard Shaw**

In every single decision you make in your life, you are creating yourself. Yes, you have a choice. Sure, there are things you can't control in this world. You can't control how others treat you. You can't control what others think of you. You can't control the lives of others. You can't make anyone else happy.

The one and only thing you can control in this life is your actions. You always have a choice. You can choose to make life sweeter. You can choose to be the best version of yourself, for yourself. You can choose to be happy.

When you choose to create the best version of yourself, you allow yourself to make the journey sweet. You give yourself the option to be happy.

On the outside, when you look at the person who appears to have everything, it may seem as if they are happy. But you never truly know. The richest person in the world may not be the wealthiest.

The only thing you know is how you feel, what you need, and what is important to you. There are many accounts in your life you can choose to fill:

Your passion account.
Your fulfillment account.
Your life experience account.
Your love account.

Choose to love yourself enough to figure out which accounts need the most attention. Start by giving your body and brain what they need to operate at your most optimal performance. When you do this you are giving yourself the opportunity to self-actualize.

Remember your body is like a car. It needs maintenance. But when you put in the effort and take the time to maintain it, your drive is smoother, there are less breakdowns and in the end you get to where you want to be so much quicker. This is the Body & Bank Connection!

# Chapter 10

# KEEP GROWING

**"One can choose to go back toward safety or forward toward growth. Growth must be chosen again and again; fear must be overcome again and again."**
**—Abraham Maslow**

One of the best things you can do for the world is share your light. To be of service to others is one of the greatest gifts you actually give to yourself. That is what this book is for me. It's a gift to you, but it is also a gift for myself. I learned so much while going through my own transformation, that I knew I couldn't just keep it for myself. It feels good to share my lessons with you, and it is my hope that you will be able to use them to make your life even better. When you do that, I know that you will then share your story with others. Because that is the thing about movements; the more momentum they gain, the more they can't help but grow.

This is a movement: The Body & Bank Connection. It's one I began to feel growth within me from the moment I felt the call to live a healthier, happier and more fulfilling life within my purpose. What is my purpose? I know that at this point you already can answer this question, but I'll share it with you again in my own words: to help those who want to be the best, healthiest, and happiest versions of themselves, not just in the work I do as a coach but in the way I lead my life.

To live within this purpose I continue to do the work. And I will keep doing this work until it is my turn to leave this earth. I keep moving. I keep growing. I have days where I fall down. I have days when I lose my drive. I have days when I get back up. But I still keep going. It's in the going that things get good, and continue to get better and better. Remember that as you finish this book and continue to move forward on your own growth journey. Keep going! Keep growing!

For this final chapter I want to pull together everything I have shared in this book and tie it into a 30-day challenge to motivate you to keep moving!

## The Body Vitality Solution

To bring it all full circle, I draw your attention back to the diagram I shared with you at the very beginning of the book. The solution to achieving both physical and financial fitness is all about the five Rs:

1. Reason
2. Resolve
3. Regime
4. Routine
5. Recovery

## Your Reason

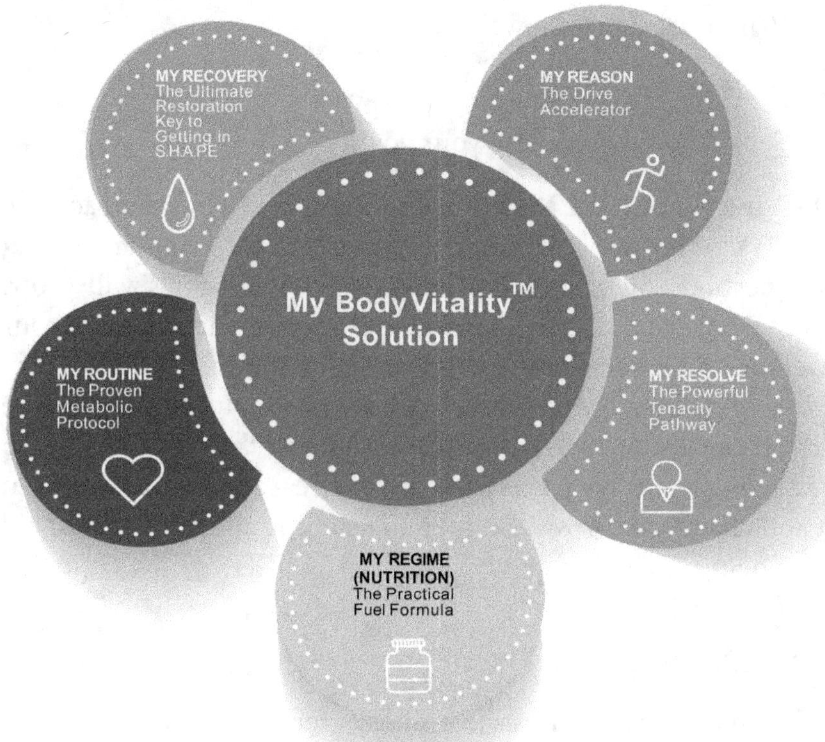


Whenever you feel like you can't keep going, come back to your reason. Ask yourself these questions now:

1.  **WHAT?**

    What are your goals?
    What are your fitness goals?
    What are your health goals?
    What are your financial goals?

2.  **WHY?**

    Why do you want to achieve your goals?
    Is it so that you can achieve a more balanced lifestyle?
    Do you want to feel better about yourself so that you are confident in all areas of your life?

3.  **WHERE?**

Where are you at now?

4.  **WHEN?**

Set a date for achieving your goal.

Does the WHAT, the WHERE, and the WHEN, help you achieve your WHY? If not, how are they out of alignment? I suggest revisiting these questions often along your journey. Your goals will grow. Where you are at will grow. I imagine if you were to compare your answers to these questions in chapter 1 to your answers now, they are already different. More knowledge allows you to see things more clearly. It can send you in a direction you never thought possible. So always, always, always come back to your reason. Know that it can shift and change and grow. Be open to listening and letting go of old ways of being.

## Your Resolve

When it comes to your resolve, always remember the 4 Cs:

1.  **Commitment**
2.  **Challenges**
3.  **Coaching**
4.  **Changes**

It is your commitment to face the challenges head on, to seek coaching when you need help, and to embrace the changes you need to make in your lifestyle that will lead you down the Powerful Tenacity Pathway.

When you resolve to achieve something, your tenacity gives you the strength to hold on. Your commitment to yourself and your goals will help you to choose the right support (coaching), to help you navigate the challenges and ultimately accept the changes you need to make to achieve your goals. Once you fully embrace the 4 Cs in your process you will have officially embarked on the Powerful

Tenacity Pathway. And let me tell you, once you are on this path you will feel the pull to succeed. You will have entered into the next phase of your development, and even though some days you may feel like it would be easier to turn back, your resolve won't let you.

Without the resolve, every obstacle you meet along the way will be an excuse to abandon or turn back from your journey. However with resolve, every obstacle will present itself as a reason to dig deeper within yourself for a solution to that puzzle and turn that struggle into vitamins to nourish you, to condition you and inspire you to grow.

## Your Regime

Make it easy for yourself to succeed in both your health and fitness goals. I'm bringing back my tip on meal prep from chapter 5, just in case you needed a reminder. This is such a simple thing and it will help you stick to your healthy eating goals. Remember you are a Ferrari! Give yourself the fuel you need to operate at your best!

### Meal Prep

DO THIS ONE THING AND I GUARANTEE YOU WILL SUCCEED!

I am not kidding. Set yourself up for success by preparing ahead of time. The easiest way to fail at creating healthier eating habits is to not be prepared for those moments when you're really hungry. Sometimes the thought of prepping food for the entire week can seem either overwhelming or boring.

I have a system that is easy, takes very little time, and ensures that the food you have made for yourself is always fresh.

First of all, I don't prep for the entire week at once. I prep meals on Sunday and Wednesday. Begin by choosing 2 days of the week that work best for your schedule.

Think about your food in terms of the three macro nutrients I talked about above:

**Protein** – pick 3 or 4 that you enjoy the most that you can rotate through

**Carbs** – choose 2 to 3 good carbs

**Fats** – this is flexible

On Sunday (or whatever day you choose for day 1), prepare at least 2 proteins and 2 carbs. Portion them out into meals for the next four days. Also portion out some healthy snacks that you can take with you on the go. Peanuts, for example, are a good healthy fat and a great snack.

On Wednesday (or whatever day you choose for day 2), prepare 2 different proteins and 2 carbs as well as your snacks.

If you find you get bored with the food you prepped and you have time one day to make yourself a healthy meal, don't fret! Just put your prepped meal in the freezer and save it for one of those days when you may not have as much prep time as you need.

## Your Routine

Trust the Proven Metabolic Protocol. It works! I know because I've both experienced it and witnessed it. Here's a quick recap on why it works:

**So, what is the Proven Metabolic Protocol?**

This is based on proven effectiveness in enhancing your metabolism, from research and studies.

In simple terms, they are short workouts, approximately 20 minutes or less, that can be done anywhere. Instead of having to go to the gym, you can simply get up in the morning and work out before you get ready for the rest of your day. No packing a bag. No leaving extra time for travel. No fussing with having to get ready for work in a crowded change room. No worrying about how much time you're wasting on these things that don't need to be done.

Get up.
Work out.
Feel good.
Get energized.
Let this one small change impact your life as a whole!

The benefits:

1.  **It's efficient** – Your workout is designed for you to achieve the maximum results in the least amount of time.

2.  **Your heart is healthier** – During these quick workouts you strengthen your heart.

3.  **Anti-aging** – It helps slow the signs of aging.

4.  **You reap the rewards right away!**

5.  **Helps balance hormones** – Reduces the production of ghrelin, the hunger hormone.

6.  **There are no barriers to achieving your goals** – Not having to depend on machinery, you can work out anytime anywhere, making it easy!

7.  **Blood-sugar balance** – Studies have shown there are benefits to blood flow and vessel dilation.

8.  **Lose weight, not muscle** – This type of physical activity promotes muscle growth!

## Your Recovery

This one is so important. If you don't give your body time to recover, you won't reach your goals. It is that simple! Pay just as much attention to your recovery as you do your workout.

If you get stuck on this one, all you have to do is remember one simple word: SHAPE! Yes, one of the key components to getting into shape in all areas of your life is restoration. And if you remember the element of shape, you will have the Ultimate Restoration Key at your fingertips:

1.  **S** – Sleep
2.  **H** – Hydrate
3.  **A** – Air
4.  **P** – Period
5.  **E** – Energy

## Your Finances

Remember to get your finances in shape too!

We've talked about how important it is to pay yourself first. If you've done this and you've invested well, shift from actively receiving to passively receiving income. In a way this is like breathing life into your investments and letting them use the energy you've given them to work for you.

Rest and let the money flow. Yes, this can happen for you, just as it has for so many others, but as I've said before: It takes time! If you start investing now in your long-term financial health, there will be a moment when you can shift from active income generation to passive income generation. Start getting your finances in shape now so they will one day work for you, even while you sleep.

Remember to make a plan! Once you have your financial statement and your cash flow, the plan is key! Your financial statement helps you see where you are at. Your cash flow is your day-to-day awareness of where your money is going. With this knowledge in hand you can begin to decrease your liabilities and increase your assets.

Again, your plan should be specific to you. Reaching your financial goals is a personal journey, and your plan should reflect that.

One strategy I teach my clients that has been very effective in paying down debt in the shortest possible time is the Snowball Debt Re-Payment Strategy. This is effective if you owe more than one account. The strategy begins by paying off the smallest debt while paying minimum payments on larger ones. Once the first debt is paid off, then you roll over that payment to the next, and so on and so forth. In theory the amounts available for repayment will grow quickly as you get towards the larger debt, like a snowball rolling downhill.

Below are the steps in the Snowball Debt Re-Payment Strategy:

1. List all debts you owe in ascending order from smallest balance to the largest.

2. Pay the minimum payment plus some extra cash you can afford towards the smallest debt until it is paid off.

3. Pay the minimum payment on every other debt.

4. Once a debt is paid off, add the old minimum payment (plus any extra amount available) from the first debt to the minimum payment on the second smallest debt, and apply the new sum to repaying the second smallest debt.

5. Repeat until all debts are paid in full.

## Your Life!

**"Even though our time in this life is temporary, if we live well enough, our legacy will last forever."**

**—Idowu Koyenikan**

One last reminder before I send you off to complete an amazing 30 day challenge that puts you on the path to achieving all of your fitness and financial goals:

## IT'S ALL ABOUT FULFILLMENT

Give yourself the tools you need to achieve both your physical and financial goals and you will begin to see massive shifts in all areas of your life! You will feel happier. You will be able to address challenges more productively. You'll start playing bigger and living life more fully. Your confidence will soar. Yes, this sounds too good to be true. I promise you that it is not. I promise if you adopt these principles and apply them to your life, you will see results!

1.  Just like exercise routines are not the means to the end, but rather the means to all of the benefits from exercise, this goes for financial discipline too. What you can achieve with your fitness goals you can also achieve with your financial goals.

2.  You don't just complete one workout and expect to receive all of the benefits. You need to be consistent and include it as a part of your routine to see those gains, which is the same for your finances. Finances require consistent discipline, and over time will not only get easier but the results will be sweeter too. It's always harder to lose that extra weight than it is to maintain a lower weight. In the same way it's harder to pay off debt than it is to maintain a debt-free life.

3.  Just like making exercise a habit, thereby requiring less effort or will power on your part, making good financial practices a habit too will help you not have to put much effort in the future. A couple easy ones are: scheduling some time a week dedicated to your finances, and automating your payments and savings.

## 30 Day Body and Bank Transformation Challenge

**"By a mile it's a trial but by an inch it's a cinch."**

**—Zig Ziglar**

As the saying goes, you don't have to be great to start but you have to start to be great, so we will begin by stacking daily disciplines for 30 days. The idea is that, as we repeat these disciplines, they will then translate into habits and it's these seemingly small wins that will then compound into major wins over time . . .

**Day 1** – Schedule some time to reflect on your current reality in both your fitness and your finances. You can take as little or as much time as you need. Establishing your own awareness of the truth is your starting point. It allows you to get clarity on what you need to change.

**Day 2** – Take some time to write about what your ideal fitness and finance scenarios look like. Really get into it.

**Day 3** – Reflect on your writing from day 1 and day 2. Where are the gaps? What habits are keeping you from achieving your goals? What needs to change in your current reality, to make your ideal reality an actual lived reality for you? The answers to these questions can sometimes take time. As you continue with the remainder of this challenge, continue to reflect on your answers here.

**Day 4** – Write down a list of people who you can count on to help you through this challenge. On the tough days, who can you talk to who has your back?

**Day 5** – Take your first leap! Ask yourself: What fitness mini goal am I committing to today? The great thing about creating a manageable goal that is easy to accomplish at the beginning is you set yourself up to win. You give yourself the gift of feeling accomplished. A manageable fitness goal could be taking a 20min walk at lunch, or walking up the stairs instead of riding the lift.

**Day 6** – What money mini goal am I committing to today? An example of a manageable goal would be opening or looking at savings accounts, or setting up an automated direct transfer to your savings, or requesting a credit report to give you a snapshot view of your liabilities, or even taking 5 minutes to look over your online account spending for the past week.

**Day 7** – Look back to the list you created on day 4. Having had a few more days to reflect, is there anyone on that list who you could ask to be your accountability partner? Who would be the best person on that list to keep you on track? If you can't think of anyone who would be a great fit, think outside of your current community. Maybe it is time to hire someone to help.

**Day 8** – Today, make one small habit change that will bring you closer to your ideal reality. It can be anything, from waking up 5 minutes early to stretch when you get out of bed, to packing a lunch rather than buying it. Big changes begin with each small step.

**Day 9** – What is your money story? Today, work on gaining more awareness about your money beliefs. Are they coming from a scarcity narrative or from an abundance narrative? Understanding this is key, because beliefs are the major drivers to how we relate to money. To get awareness, you need to understand how you perceive money. Do you regard money as a tool in your arsenal that brings all these benefits or do you regard it through a negative lens, that it's only available for the lucky few?

**Day 10** – Today take stock of your support system. Is your social support propping you up and challenging you to get better, or bringing you down? Ensure you have a support system that fosters an environment of growth and gets you out of your comfort zone. If you haven't done so already, decide on an accountability partner and make sure they are on board. This is one of the most important steps, which is why I keep coming back to it. If there is anyone who is unsupportive of the changes you want to make, it may be time to limit the amount of time you spend with them. I know this can be difficult. You might have that great friend who always wants to hit the bar for a few pints after work, or even a family member who always pushes you to eat in a way that doesn't work for you. Find ways to limit their influence on your lifestyle choices.

**Day 11** – Today take time to journal what you eat and how you feel after. Again, awareness in the beginning. Without it, how will you know what to change! Be honest in your journaling. Make sure to record everything.

**Day 12** – It's time to understand where your money is going. Take a look at your expenses for the past week. Are there any surprises? It's a good financial habit to periodically take audit to ensure you know what is coming in and going out.

**Day 13** – Schedule a meal prep for the week to include the 3 key macro nutrients of carbs, protein and dietary fats.

**Day 14** – What are your go-to snacks? Are they healthy? If not, write a list of healthier go-to snacks and stock your home with those. Remove the unhealthy ones from your home.

**Day 15** – Today's task is an easy one. Take a look at your next few days and schedule a good chunk of time, like an hour or two, to go over your monthly income and expenses. It's time to get a very clear picture of what your financial health is at the moment.

**Day 16** – Get walking! Take a 20-minute walk today and schedule 2 more to happen within the next week.

**Day 17** – Use the knowledge that you've gained in your work so far to set up an automatic transfer from your regular account to a savings/investment account.

**Day 18** – Today schedule and put in a 10-20min workout— If you need some help deciding how you want to work out, head to my website at www.bodyandbankconnection.com for some same samples.

**Day 19** – Schedule in 5 minutes a day, starting today, to continue to review your finances. I know you may not see any drastic changes, but the more opportunities you take to see the reality of what is happening, the clearer you'll get on what you need to do moving forward.

**Day 20** – Answer this: How many hours of sleep did you get last night? Do you feel rested? How does this compare to an average night for you? Do you think there are some changes that need to be made here?

**Day 21** – Keep a record of how much water you drink today. At the end of the day, take note of whether you are getting enough or if you need to drink more.

**Day 22** – Look back at the work you've done to understand what your current financial picture is. How much can you set aside on a monthly basis to pay towards your credit cards or loans to reduce those liabilities and increase your assets?

**Day 23** – Again, have a look at your financial situation and think about how much you can commit on a monthly basis to start growing your nest egg. If this is a difficult question to answer, it might be time to think about getting some financial advice.

**Day 24** – Today, take time to consciously get some active rest and breathe. It's when we rest and breathe that all the magic happens. You've been working hard both mentally and physically. Give yourself the break you need today.

**Day 25** – What new money or fitness discipline will you introduce today? This could be adding in another 20min walk, increasing your water intake, understanding what current expenses can you cut out, bringing a packed lunch to work, or starting to read some financial literature.

**Day 26** – Sometimes in order to create lasting change you need to get out of your comfort zone. What is one thing you can do today to push yourself? It can be anything. Sing out loud in the shower. Put on some fun music and dance around your house.

Talk to someone new. Wear that bright colored shirt that you love but have been too shy to wear.

**Day 27** –  Reflect on your current daily fitness routine. With this challenge you've been getting more active. You've been changing your habits. What is the most important discipline with your fitness you can work on this week?

**Day 28** –  Reflect on your current daily financial routine. With this challenge you've been getting more clear. You've been changing your habits. What is the most important financial discipline you can work on this week?

**Day 29** –  Write down three things that went well with your health and fitness yesterday and 3 things you can do better today.

**Day 30** –  I left the biggest one for last. This is the question that will ensure you achieve both your fitness and financial goals. ARE YOU PAYING YOURSELF FIRST?

## Need Some Help?

Remember that you never have to do anything alone. If you feel like you are about to give up, reach out to a friend, a family member, your accountability partner, or hire a coach. If you'd like to learn more about my services or schedule a chat, check out my website: **www.bodyandbankconnection.com**